D1446838

PIONEERS OF MEDICINE

AND THEIR IMPACT ON

TUBERCULOSIS

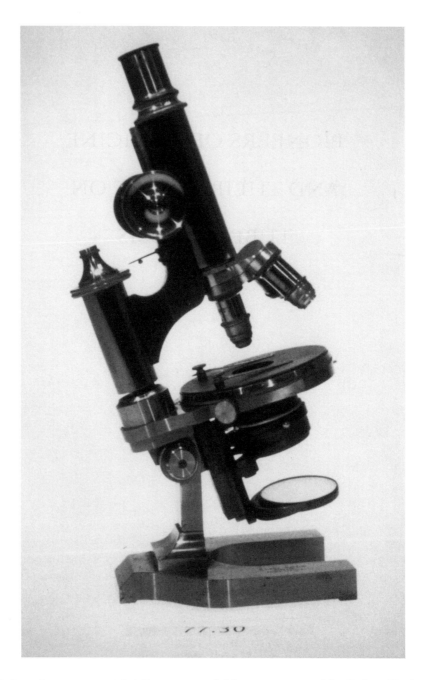

Leitz microscope, 1896. Microscopes of this type were used by Robert Koch and his associates. Dittrick Center for Medical History, Case Western Reserve University, Cleveland, Ohio.

PIONEERS OF MEDICINE AND THEIR IMPACT ON TUBERCULOSIS

THOMAS M. DANIEL

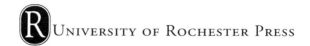
Ⓡ UNIVERSITY OF ROCHESTER PRESS

First published 2000
by the University of Rochester Press

The University of Rochester Press is an imprint of
Boydell & Brewer, Inc.
668 Mt. Hope Avenue, Rochester, NY 14620, USA
and of Boydell & Brewer, Ltd.
P.O. Box 9, Woodbridge, Suffolk 1P12 3DF, UK

hard cover: ISBN 1–58046–067–4

Library of Congress Cataloging-in-Publication Data

Daniel, Thomas M.
    Pioneers in medicine and their impact on tuberculosis /
Thomas M. Daniel.
        p. cm.
    Includes bibliographical references and index.
    ISBN 1–58046–067–4 (alk. paper)
        1. Tuberculosis—History.   2. Medical scientists—Biography.
    I. Title.

RC310.D36 2000
616.9′95′009—dc 21   00–062850

British Library Cataloguing-in-Publication Data
A catalogue record for this book is available from the British Library

Designed and typeset by ISIS-1 Corporation
Printed in the United States of America
This publication is printed on acid-free paper

*For the many predoctoral
and postdoctoral students
who have made my life exciting.*

Contents

Illustrations

Portraits

Figures

Tables

Introduction

Pioneers in Medicine and Their Effect on Tuberculosis is about six men whose lives spanned nearly two centuries. They were pioneers who moved into the van far beyond their contemporaries in medicine to lead in establishing new fields of scientific endeavor. They were truly innovative thinkers.

The book traces the origins and early evolution of six fields of medical science. The men profiled here lived in remarkable times that saw the emergence of separate scientific medical disciplines. During these times, the medicine we know today emerged from the chrysalis of mysticism and metamorphosed into an evidence-based discipline. Each of the six pioneers described in this book was one of the early founders of his discipline.

This book emphasizes the interrelatedness of all scientific medical thought. It is a paradox that scientists and medical practitioners find it necessary to focus and limit their efforts in order to build the expertise upon which advances in understanding are built, yet knowledge does not prosper in insular environments. Despite currently increasing specialization not only of medical practitioners but also of research scientists, new knowledge requires a solid foundation of previously established science. As knowledge in a medical discipline expands, it requires more and more links both to its own history and to other similarly evolving disciplines. The history of medicine is important to its present and future; the breadth of medicine is important to its focus and precision.

Throughout history, tuberculosis has been at or near the top of the list of infectious illness that have plagued humankind. This pervasive disease has had a central position not only in causing illness but also in challenging medical scientists to understand it—and, in so doing, to understand further all of human health and illness. The six pioneers whose stories are told in this volume worked on tuberculosis. For some, it was the major focus of their efforts; for others, one of a number of interests. Two of them actually suffered from the disease themselves. Tuberculosis provides a central theme for this book, a theme that unites the work of these six pioneers, a theme that serves well to illustrate the relatedness of scientific medical disciplines. The book is not specifically about tuberculosis, yet that disease is never far from its pages, just as it was never far from the lives of these six pioneers.

The physicians, biomedical scientists, and other health professionals who are my present and future colleagues in the crusade to conquer tuberculosis will likely find that knowledge of their intellectual origins enriches their present science and art. Historians and general readers interested in the history of medical science may find this book of interest, and for them I have included a glossary.

For some who read this book, tuberculosis may be at the center of their careers, as it was for mine during nearly four decades. For others, tuberculosis may be a nearly unknown disease. Thus, the background of this book's readers may be disparate, and this consideration has dictated some of its organization. The first three chapters, Part 1, are intended to bring all readers to a common level of understanding of tuberculosis, preparing them to understand the work of the six medical pioneers described in Part 2 and the central position of tuberculosis both in their work and in the history of medical science. The first chapter highlights the role of this disease in the evolution of scientific medical knowledge; the second describes the pathogenesis of tuberculosis; the third its secular epidemiology. Part 2 of the book presents six pioneers of medical science. For each, the times in which he worked and his life is described. For each, his accomplishments are considered both in light of his own times and present knowledge. Part 3 is a brief reflective epilogue.

This book has its origins in my earlier book presenting tuberculosis to general readers (*Captain of Death: The Story of Tuberculosis*, University of Rochester Press, 1997). As I researched that book, I was repeatedly impressed by the rigor of thought and quality of investigation that marked the work of some of the scientists whose contributions I described. They needed a better and deeper look, I thought. I chose the six men upon whom this book focuses because each of them was truly a founding pioneer of a separate discipline. The unfolding story of their lives during two hundred years is more than the story of six men. It is the story of the evolution of much of modern medicine.

I am not a historian. I am, I believe, an interpreter of medical history. Almost all of this work relies on secondary sources—on previously published biographies and biographical articles, which I have carefully referenced in my end notes. However, I have read all of the scientific papers referenced in this book. These papers constitute the bulk of the output of these pioneers, and they are primary source material for an analysis of the importance of these men. Moreover, I have read them not as a biographer but as a fellow scientist and practitioner of medicine, drawing on my own background and experience as an investigator, physician, and student of disease—including tuberculosis—with each of these roles.

Acknowledgments

I have received the help of many persons in preparing this book. First I wish to acknowledge the staff and librarians of the Cleveland Health Sciences Library, including the Allen Medical Library with its extraordinary historical collection. Next, I am grateful to the Center for International Health of the Case Western Reserve University School of Medicine, where I have been provided with office space, facilities, and support as an emeritus professor. There are many professional colleagues with whom I have discussed either formally or informally various parts of the content of this book. When appropriate, I have noted these sources in end notes. Particularly important were Jack Gwaltney of the University of Virginia, who provided me with interesting biographical information about Wade Hampton Frost, and Margaret Oxtoby and Tom Flynn of the New York State Health Department and Dickerson Library, who provided me with access to material about Hermann Biggs. The biographical accounts of the pioneers included in this book are greatly enriched by the portraits drawn by Theresa Chung. Marlene Faust and Laurin Kasehagen of the Case Western Reserve University Center for Tuberculosis Research were helpful to me in scanning text from scientific papers and thus saving me the effort of typing many passages quoted in this book. Finally, as with everything I write, I am grateful to my wife, Janet Daniel, who has read the entire text and provided me with corrections of my grammatical and typographical errors and also stimulation, encouragement, an occasional pointed criticism—and love.

PART I

Medicine and the White Plague

"The time has come," the Walrus said,
      "To talk of many things:
Of shoes—and ships—and sealing wax—
      "Of Cabbages—and kings—
And why the sea is boiling hot—
      And whether pigs have wings."
                              Lewis Carroll
            "The Walrus and the Carpenter"

1

Medical History and Tuberculosis— The Warp and the Weft

The warp threads of medical history began to roll off the loom beam as early as we know of human thought. The tapestry woven on them continues to the present and will continue as long as people inhabit the earth. For there is nothing as precious to us as our well-being, and society has always called forth and will always call forth its brightest minds and deftest workers to add to the cloth of medical knowledge.

Throughout history, many of the weft threads of medicine have been colored by tuberculosis, the dread disease. Not surprisingly, the succession of shamans, priests, physicians, and other healers who assumed responsibility for the care of people directed its attention to this illness, for the white plague was then and is today an important disease. Common throughout much of history, tuberculosis remains of interest to biomedical scientists in the modern world of its diminishing incidence because it serves as the prototype for infections mediated by intracellular pathogens and as a paradigm for cell-mediated immune mechanisms. As medical science has advanced from mystical incantations to molecular biology, tuberculosis has marched in the van of its progress.

Today, those of us who live in prosperous, technologically advanced societies scarcely think of tuberculosis as an important disease. However, those of us who live in impoverished, developing countries know that the Captain of Death is not far from us and are not surprised to learn that it has killed more of us than any other infection. Considered in the context of history, however, even those of us who are fortunate to have put tuberculosis behind us are not far removed from it. A century ago, it was one of our leading causes of death; many of us remember forebear who died of "TB" or who "cured" at a "san." It should not come as a surprise to us, then, that so much of the fabric of our knowledge of disease and disease processes is woven of fibers from the study of tuberculosis.

If we contemplate infectious diseases, then we can examine an unrolling tapestry from (1) the dawning of concepts of infection to (2) the recognition of pathogenic microorganisms to (3) the modern sciences of public health and epidemiology to (4) the study of immunologically mediated host resistance to (5) the new scientific arena of molecular biology. As our knowledge in these fields advanced, it was repeatedly and inseparably interwoven with our knowledge of tuberculosis. Let us take a closer look; let us consider each of these five fields of biomedical endeavor.

Concepts of Infection

Hippocrates, known to every physician for the oath attributed to him, was perhaps the greatest of the Asclepiads from the Greek island of Kos. His dates are usually given as 460 to 370 B.C.E., at the dawning of the great classic era of Greece. His medicine was oriented to his patients, with systematic observation of ill persons forming the basis of diagnosis. Moreover, he introduced ethical concepts into medical practice that remain the basis for current standards.

Hippocrates described epidemic diseases in Athens, considering, phthisis, pulmonary tuberculosis, the most important of them:

> Early in the beginning of spring, and through the summer, and towards winter, many of those who had been long gradually declining, took to bed with symptoms of phthisis; in many cases formerly of a doubtful character the disease then became confirmed; in these the constitution inclined to the phthisical. Many, and in fact, the most of them died. . . . Consumption was the most considerable of the diseases which then prevailed, and the only one which proved fatal to many persons.[1]

Hippocrates did not, however, consider tuberculosis infectious. His contemporary, Thucydides, who was not a physician, also wrote of epidemics in Athens and did. The Roman physician, Galen, may have understood that some diseases, including tuberculosis, were infectious.

It was the "black death," bubonic plague, that made it dramatically obvious that certain diseases were infectious in nature. An ancient disease described in the Old Testament and responsible for periodic regional epidemics throughout human history and across the globe, plague crept out of Asia in the 1330s and 1340s, carried by fleas traveling on rats along trade routes. Then, in the late 1340s, it stormed across Europe, killing one-quarter to one-third of the population in about three years. Some have estimated that it killed as much as half of the population. While various causes were assigned to the plague by civil authorities, it was widely assumed by the populace to be contagious, and when possible, victims were shunned and isolated. At the end of the fourteenth century, major port cities of the Mediterranean enacted the first quarantine laws for ships; the word "quarantine" derives from the Italian "quarantina," meaning forty days, the usual period of detention. It was clear to everyone that ships or something associated with them were major vectors.

In the sixteenth century, the Swiss mystic known as Paracelsus, whose actual name was Aureolus Theophrastus Bombastus von Hohenheim, had his ideas about medicine firmly rooted in alchemy and astrology. He also may have been among the first to understand the infectious nature of some diseases. His contemporary, Hieronymus Fracastorius Veronensis, is generally credited with the earliest clear elucidation of the infectious nature of diseases. In 1584 he wrote:

> The fundamental differences of all contagions are seen to be three in number: those infecting by contact alone, those only by contact and leaving fomites by which they are contagious such as scabies, phthisis, itch, baldness, elephantiasis and others of this sort . . . [2]

He continued, indicating that among contagious diseases he intended to include those transmissible at a distance. Interestingly, he attributed all such transmission to fomites, not apparently recognizing airborne infections. And pulmonary tuberculosis, phthisis in the terminology of his day, joined such maladies as baldness, scabies, and itch on his list of contagious diseases.

The concepts of infectiousness that had germinated in Italy did not take root elsewhere. In 1836 Frédéric Chopin and George Sand went to Mallorca hoping for amelioration of Chopin's tuberculosis in the tropical climate of that Mediterranean Island. To their surprise and dismay, they were soon expelled from Palma by the local citizens who considered tuberculosis infectious. Tuberculosis was considered an inherited and noncontagious condition in Northern Europe at that time. Sand later wrote of this episode:

> [W]e had succeeded in settling down at Majorca, a magnificent place, but inhospitable to the utmost degree. At the end of a month, poor Chopin, who had always been coughing from the time we left Paris, fell more seriously ill, so that we had to call in one, two, three doctors, each more asinine than the others, who went about the island saying that the patient was in the last stage of consumption. This caused great consternation, phthisis being extremely rare in those latitudes, and, moreover, considered contagious! Added to this were the egotism, the cowardice, the want of feeling, and the bad faith of the inhabitants. We were looked upon as pestiferous, and, worse, as heathens, for we did not attend mass. The landlord of the little cottage that we had hired ejected us brutally, and wanted to bring an action against us in order to compel us to whitewash his house, which he pretended was infected. Had he succeeded, the native jurisprudence would have completely skinned us![3]

The great British surgeon, John Hunter, inoculated himself with syphilis in May 1767, thinking that he was merely dealing with gonorrhea, and this unhappy experiment proved to be a landmark in the demonstration that some diseases could be transmitted from one individual to another. Theophile Laennec inadvertently inoculated his finger with tuberculosis while performing an autopsy in 1803 (Chapter 4). While Laennec probably did not draw the obvious conclusion from his accident, he did attempt to disinfect the wound at the time. Forty years later, Oliver Wendell Holmes and Ignaz P. Semmelweis campaigned for hygiene and physician hand-washing as means of preventing the transmission of puerperal sepsis. In 1864 Casimir Davaine transmitted anthrax from animal to animal. One year later, the weft of the tapestry was again colored by tuberculosis, when Jean-Antoine Villemin transmitted tuberculosis to a rabbit by inoculating the animal with material from a pulmonary cavity of a man who had died of tuberculosis. A control animal, housed with the inoculated one, did not develop tuberculosis. Villemin clearly understood the implications of his experiment and unequivocally considered tuberculosis an infectious disease.[4] In 1868, an English physician named William Budd, argued that tuberculosis was spread from person to person and "that the tuberculous matter itself is (or includes) the specific morbific matter of the disease, and constitutes the material by which phthisis is propagated from one person to another and disseminated through society."[5]

When Robert Koch discovered the bacterial etiology of tuberculosis, little doubt could remain that this disease was infectious, although some still failed to see the obvious. In accepting the Nobel Prize in 1905, Koch recalled:

> But it was not till the tubercle bacillus was discovered that the etiology of tuberculosis was placed on a sure foundation and the conviction gained that it is not only a parasitic—i.e., an infectious—but also an avoidable disease. Even in my first publications on the etiology of tuberculosis I pointed to the dangers which arise from the dissemination of the secretions of those suffering from pulmonary phthisis containing bacilli and called for prophylactic measures against the pestilence. But my words were not attended to. The reason was that it was still too early. . . .[6]

Thus, in the late nineteenth century it had become firmly established that some diseases, prominently including tuberculosis, were infectious. The stage was set, draped in part with fabric woven of the white plague, and in subsequent years the drama of this infectivity and of efforts to prevent the spread of disease were incorporated into the tapestry of medical history with the discovery of increasing numbers of pathogenic microorganisms.

The concept that diseases could be transmitted aerially began with Koch's work on tuberculosis, but would have to await the twentieth century for its full development. Again, in his Nobel Prize acceptance Koch noted:

> At the same time, however, attention must be paid to the fact that it is not only the secretion of the lungs called sputum that is dangerous as containing bacilli, but that according to Flügge's investigations the minutest droplets of phlegm that are flung into the air by the patients when they cough and clear their throats and even when they speak also contain bacilli and can thereby cause infection.[7]

Carl Flügge, to whom Koch referred, worked at Koch's institute in Berlin. He demonstrated that dried sputum, even when ground to a fine dust, did not reach the small air spaces of the lungs where tuberculosis begins with the nidation of inhaled organisms. In the 1940s William Firth Wells and his colleagues convincingly demonstrated the role of bacteria-containing droplet nuclei in the transmission of respiratory infections; again tuberculosis was at the center of these studies.[8] Ultimately, fomites were abandoned in medical thought as important in the transmission of most respiratory infections, a concept that was finally put to rest by the work of John Chapman and Margaret Dyerly studying the children of tuberculosis patients in Texas in 1964.[9] They found that once the infectious tuberculous patient was removed from the home, infection of children ceased, even though the environment was not decontaminated. That air could continue to remain infectious far removed from the infectious source patient or long after the secretor of pathogens had left the environment became suspected in the face of spreading smallpox; it was demonstrated for tuberculosis by the studies of T. V. Hyge of transmission of infection in a Danish school room[10] and by those of Richard Riley and his colleagues of the infectiousness of tuberculosis patients in a Baltimore hospital.[11] Once again, the thread of knowledge was woven into the tapestry by the shuttle of tuberculosis.

Pathogenic Microorganisms

Anton van Leewenhoek was a Dutch lens grinder living in Delft. He made and used many simple microscopes, and with them observed bacteria scraped from his teeth, which he described in a letter written to the Royal Society of London in 1684.[12] That such small "animalcula" could be responsible for disease was not envisioned for more than forty years. Then, in 1720, Benjamin Marten, an English physician, published a remarkable book entitled, *A New Theory of Consumptions: More Especially of a Phthisis or Consumption of the Lungs*, in which he unequivocally stated that tuberculosis and other diseases, including "itch, leprosy, and venereal distemper," were caused by the animalcula described by Leewenhoek.[13] Others of that time had speculated on the relationship of Leewenhoek's minute organisms to disease, but it was Martens, writing about tuberculosis, who most clearly conceptualized it.

Knowledge of disease exploded during the nineteenth century. Among many advances in thought, the concept of infections caused by microorganisms became firmly established. Joseph Lister introduced asepsis to surgery. Louis Pasteur studied pebrine, a disease of silkworms, and concluded that it was a microbial infection. It was Robert Koch, however, first with anthrax in 1876 and then with tuberculosis in 1882, who first convincingly demonstrated the bacterial etiology of human diseases. In the process, he defined the criteria for such a demonstration, criteria now known as Koch's postulates. More than that, in the course of his studies, Koch invented and introduced several fundamental bacteriological techniques. He made the first cultures on solid medium; without such cultures it is impossible to obtain pure cultures of organisms from clinical material, a sine qua non of both clinical and investigational bacteriology. Koch was a pioneer in the use of oil-immersion microscopy. He took the first photomicrographs of bacteria. He introduced novel staining techniques for differentiating bacteria. He made major contributions to techniques for sterilization. He is justifiably considered the father of the science of bacteriology, and the primitive laboratory in which he conducted his studies of tuberculosis was surely the obstetrical delivery room for this discipline. Returning to the weaving metaphor, Koch's work, described in Chapter 5, wove the tubercle bacillus brilliantly into the central images of the tapestry of the history of infectious diseases.

Among the giants of the early days of bacteriology was Theobald Smith, a man whom we will consider again as we discuss immunity. Smith was the individual who described *Mycobacterium bovis*, distinguishing it as the cause of tuberculosis in cattle from the human pathogen, *M. tuberculosis*. Smith's effort launched a massive North American campaign to eradicate bovine tuberculosis, one of the earliest national efforts in public health. Koch vehemently resisted Smith's ideas, but the latter's arguments prevailed, and bovine tuberculosis was effectively controlled by the end of the second decade of the twentieth century.

Public Health and Epidemiology

With the modes of transmission and the causes of infectious diseases rapidly becoming apparent, societies responded by developing and institutionalizing methods for the control of these diseases. We have noted that quarantine of ships originated during the great epidemic of plague in the fourteenth century. In 1699 the Italian Republic of Lucca enacted the first laws intended to prevent the spread of tuberculosis. Physicians were required to report their consumptive patients, and those caring for such patients were "to leave the entrance open from time to time, for egress of fresh air, and to take care that the patient does not empty his sputum except in vessels of glass or glazed earthenware, and that these utensils be frequently cleansed and boiled in lye at least twice. . . ."[14] Similar laws were propagated in Spain in 1751, in Florence in 1754, and in Naples in 1792. The ostracism experienced by Frédéric Chopin and George Sand was not exceptional in Southern Europe.

Robert Koch, famous and triumphant in the wake of his dramatic presentation on the etiology of tuberculosis, was given his first professorial appointment in 1885 not in bacteriology or pathology but in hygiene (Chapter 4). While this post might not have been the one he would have selected had other options been open, he took the public health aspects of it seriously. In fact, in 1887 he rebuffed the young Elie Metchnikoff, who wished to show him his preparations demonstrating phagocytoses, by saying, "You know, I am not a specialist in microscopical anatomy; I am a hygienist."[15] Nearly twenty years later he would devote his Nobel Prize address not to bacteriology but to a status report on public health aspects of tuberculosis.

On the other side of the Atlantic Ocean, Hermann Biggs was forcing public health upon New York City, much opposed in his actions by the local physicians and newspapers (Chapter 6). Biggs much admired Koch, and he saw in the work of the German a clear mandate for the implementation of public health control measures. Early public health laws in the North American colonies had been enacted in Massachusetts and Virginia in the late seventeenth century in attempts to control the spread of smallpox. Quarantine laws followed in major port cities, especially in response to threats of imported cholera. The first American national public health law was passed when the country was less than a decade old; it authorized the president to use forces available to him to assist local authorities in enforcing their quarantine laws. State and local health boards were formed in the eighteenth and nineteenth centuries in response to threats of yellow fever, malaria, and cholera. Then, as the twentieth century dawned, Hermann Biggs marched to the fore in New

York City, required the reporting of tuberculosis, and launched campaigns to educate the public on the perils of infectious tuberculosis. Within a few years, health departments throughout the nation had followed Biggs's lead.

A remarkable public health campaign led to the virtual eradication of bovine tuberculosis and the hazard of transmission of this disease by milk early in the twentieth century.[16] Shortly after Robert Koch described tuberculin in 1890 (Chapter 5), the Danish veterinarian Bernhard Bang obtained the material and used it to tuberculin test dairy cows in Copenhagen, observing that all reactive animals had tuberculosis. One year later Leonard Pearson traveled to Germany to obtain Koch's tuberculin, which he used to test cattle in Pennsylvania, again observing that all of the reacting animals were diseased when autopsied. In the United States, the Bureau of Animal Industry tuberculin tested seventeen hundred cattle in the District of Columbia in 1909. Nineteen percent reacted and were slaughtered. Two years later, only 1.4 percent of Washington's cattle were infected, and within a decade it was apparent to all that bovine tuberculosis could be eliminated. A national campaign based on tuberculin testing and slaughter of infected animals began in 1917, and by 1940 fewer than one-half of one percent of American cattle reacted to tuberculin.

Voluntary health agencies now represent the public in many advocacy roles. They entered medical history on the weft threads of tuberculosis. The first such agency was organized in Philadelphia in 1892 under the leadership of Lawrence Flick, a visionary physician who believed that the care of indigent persons with the disease should be a public responsibility. In 1904 a Danish postal clerk suggested the sale of Christmas stamps; the practice spread rapidly through Scandinavia and then to the United States. Similar seals are now sold by several voluntary agencies to raise money for a variety of causes. Also in 1904 Edward Livingston Trudeau, best remembered as the founder of the Adirondack Cottage Sanitarium at Saranac Lake, New York, joined with Flick and others to found the National Association for the Study and Prevention of Tuberculosis, the first voluntary health agency. Raising money through the sale of Christmas Seals, it ultimately moved from tuberculosis to other respiratory diseases including asthma and cigarette-related illnesses, changing its name to the American Lung Association.

Hand in hand with the applied discipline of public health grew the more academic science of epidemiology. It also drew much of its fabric from tuberculosis, most notably in the work of Wade Hampton Frost (Chapter 8). Frost began his career in bacteriology and public health. His mathematical mind carried him into a more statistically oriented approach to disease. He became the first professor of epidemiology at the newly founded Johns Hopkins University School of Hygiene and Public Health. He, like Laennec, another of the pioneers featured in this volume, experienced tuberculosis as a patient. In his studies of tuberculosis in Tennessee, Frost introduced the use of index cases as the starting point of epidemiological investigations. Later, in his seminal study of age-specific tuberculosis mortality in Massachusetts, he introduced the use of cohort analysis to the main stream of epidemiology.

Immunologically Mediated Host Resistance

Paul Ehrlich was among those who listened to Robert Koch present his observations on the tubercle bacillus on March 26, 1882. He was profoundly impressed by Koch's work and is quoted as having later said, "I hold that evening to be the most important experience of my scientific life."[17] Ehrlich recognized the acid-fast property of tubercle bacilli and thus improved Koch's staining technique; he used the new stain to find tubercle bacilli in his own sputum. Among his greatest contributions was the arsenical Salvarsan. Developed as a treatment for trypanosomiasis, it was efficacious against syphilis and stands in history as the first effective antimicrobial agent. Ehrlich received the Nobel Prize, not for one of his many enduring discoveries, but for his side chain theory of immune reactions, a now long-discarded hypothesis.

Where did the science of immunology begin? When was it recognized that humans could acquire protective immunity against pathogenic organisms?[18] Perhaps our story should begin with variolation, the practice of scratching a small amount of smallpox (variola) scabrous material into the skin of the forearm or other site of a susceptible individual. In this way, a limited case of smallpox was induced, protecting the individual from further, more devastating disease. The practice began in Asia and made its way to Europe and North America in the eighteenth century. In 1796, William Jenner introduced vaccination, using scabrous material from the lesions of cow pox (vaccinia), because he had observed that persons who had had cow pox did not contract smallpox. Louis Pasteur's rabies vaccination followed in 1885. Against this background, it is not surprising that Koch sought to induce immunity with products of the tubercle bacilli, thus hoping to ameliorate the established disease (Chapter 5). That he failed is unfortunate, but for his time his efforts represented an important advance in immunological thought.

Theobald Smith, the person who distinguished *M. bovis* from *M. tuberculosis*, is the individual who first observed that protection against infection could be conferred with the serum of an immune animal. This observation led directly to the development by Emil von Behring, working in Koch's institute, of life-saving diphtheria antitoxin; for this work Behring received the first awarded Nobel Prize in Medicine or Physiology. In fact, antiserum treatment of tuberculosis was tried and embraced briefly by physicians before it was recognized as ineffective. Clemens von Pirquet (Chapter 7), remembered in the tuberculosis community for having developed the tuberculin skin test and among allergists for having coined the term "allergy," first described serum sickness and, drawing upon his bedside observations, recognized the anamnestic "booster" response.

With antibodies now firmly established as the prime mediators of immune protection, Merrill Chase was surprised to find in 1941 that lymphocytes and not serum transferred the cutaneous reactions to certain chemicals that he was studying under the disbelieving eyes of Karl Landsteiner. After Landsteiner's death, Chase began working with René DuBos, whose major interest was tuberculosis, and he found that lymphocytes were the mediators of tuberculin reactions. We now know that certain classes of lymphocytes—T lymphocytes—are the critical elements in these delayed, cell-mediated responses.

The tapestry of the history of immunology was further enriched by weft threads contributed by G. Pearmain and his New Zealand colleagues and Robert Schrek who independently and essentially simultaneously demonstrated in 1963 that cellular immune mechanisms could be studied *in vitro* by observing changes in the morphology of lymphocytes; today these same effects are demonstrated by measuring the incorporation of isotopically labelled thymidine into the genetic material of the cells. Another step was added when John David and Barry Bloom, again independently and simultaneously, demonstrated migration inhibition factor, the first of many cytokines to be discovered. Both David and Bloom continued their interest in tuberculosis and made numerous further contributions to our understanding of that disease.

Finally, one cannot leave the subject of host resistance without noting that native resistance, which is not mediated by immune mechanisms, is also of great importance. Max Lurie became ill with tuberculosis while a senior medical student at Cornell University in 1921.[19] With this event, the Captain of Death had struck his family in each of four successive generations. Lurie went to the National Jewish Hospital in Colorado to "cure" and to pursue a residency in experimental pathology, which he thought would be less arduous than one in a clinical field. Small wonder that he chose to study familial aspects of susceptibility to tuberculosis. Lurie bred rabbits, successfully developing families susceptible to or resistant to inhaled challenges of tubercle bacilli. Later, he developed inbred strains of guinea pigs, including strains that became important to experimental oncologists because tumors could be transplanted in them. An entire science has now developed around the use of inbred mice and other laboratory animals. Its origins were woven into the fabric of medical history by Max Lurie's work on tuberculosis with rabbits.

Molecular Biology

Biomedical knowledge advances exponentially. If our metaphoric tapestry began on a primitive back-strap loom or on warp threads wound around two poles staked on the ground before advancing to a giant vertical Gobelin loom, it is now being woven faster than the eye can follow by the fly shuttle of a powered, computer-controlled, Jacquard loom. And the advancing edge is dominated by molecular biology. Where does tuberculosis stand in that science? Scarcely in the van. First of all, rapidly declining tuberculosis incidence in North America and Europe led to complacency and an insidious attitude that further knowledge was not needed—that the tools needed to control or eliminate the White

Plague were all already at hand. Public funding for tuberculosis research dwindled and corporations poured their developmental money into diseases offering potentially brighter fiscal rewards. Young scientists were not attracted to the field. Also of great importance was the tubercle bacillus itself. One must remember that the generation time of *M. tuberculosis* is about twenty-two hours. Compare that with twenty minutes for *Escherichia coli*. Who would not choose to do experiments that could be completed in hours rather than weeks? Moreover, work with virulent *M. tuberculosis* requires a P-3 containment facility; *E. coli* can be handled anywhere. Why would one choose to work with such an inconvenient organism?

Some did choose.[20] Richard Young at the Whitehead Institute developed a DNA expression library for *M. tuberculosis*, allowing the identification of many mycobacterial genes and the production of mycobacterial antigens in *E. coli*. The genes for resistance to drugs used for treating tuberculosis were identified. Jack Crawford studied mycobacterial plasmids, relating them to virulence in some organisms, and William Jacobs combined plasmids with mycobacteriophages to create vectors for implanting genes into mycobacteria. Polymerase chain reaction (PCR) amplification and restriction fragment length polymorphism analysis (DNA fingerprinting) of mycobacteria became possible with the identification by Kathleen Eisenach of a genetic transposon designated IS-6110. This ability was used by Peter Small and others to trace the spread of tuberculosis through communities and by Pablo Bifani, Bonnie Plikaytis, Barry Kreisworth, and their collaborators to elucidate the evolutionary genealogy of the multidrug-resistant strain W that killed many persons in New York City and the New York State penitentiary system in the early 1990s. Finally, in 1998, the entire genome of a virulent strain of *M. tuberculosis* was sequenced by an international team led by Stewart Cole. From this, the genes for drug resistance have been identified, and the first inklings of what makes tubercle bacilli virulent have appeared.

Unfortunately, it required the resurgence of tuberculosis in the United States during the decade beginning in 1984 to stimulate renewed interest in this disease and attract additional research dollars and research scientists to its study. One must hope that the turn-around that has been accomplished in American tuberculosis control is not once again followed by complacency toward research on the world's number-one infectious disease killer. Tuberculosis, much of it drug-resistant, continues to rage in Eastern Europe, Africa, Asia, and parts of South America. Tuberculosis rides on the coattails of AIDS, and in Africa it is the number-one opportunistic infection of HIV-infected persons. There is much warp remaining on the beam, much tapestry remaining to weave.

2

The Pathogenesis and Natural History
of Tuberculosis

Igor Stravinsky was one of the most creative musical composers the world has known. Tuberculosis stalked him throughout his life.[1] Born in 1882, he developed tuberculous pleurisy with effusion as a teenager in 1895. As is usually the case, he recovered from this illness, only to relapse with pulmonary tuberculosis in 1939. He improved with rest, but continued to have pulmonary symptoms. Stravinsky's first wife and daughter both died of tuberculosis, perhaps infected by him. In 1969, the great composer again suffered a clinical relapse. He was treated and regained his health. He lived two more years, dying in 1971 at the age of eighty-nine.

Samuel Johnson, a literary giant of his day, was only two and one-half years old in 1712 when he was taken to London to be touched by Queen Anne in hopes that his scrofula—tuberculous cervical adenitis—might be cured.[2] In fact, the royal touch was not remarkably successful, and Johnson carried disfiguring fistulae and scars throughout his life, concealing them by wearing a scarf. Yet he did not develop pulmonary tuberculosis.

Amedeo Modigliani blazed across the world of canvas-painted images with a fiery passion that set the art community of the early twentieth century aflame. At age thirty-five and at the zenith of his immense popularity, he developed tuberculous meningitis, rapidly succumbing to this illness in 1920.[3]

As a young man Galen Clark was plagued by tuberculosis. His wife died of it. After a major hemoptysis in 1855, he sought relief in the Sierra Mountains of California.[4] There, in the Yosemite Valley and among groves of giant redwood trees, he was joined by John Muir, whose life would also be touched by tuberculosis.[5] Clark regained his health, and the lives and work of Clark and Muir as naturalists led to the widespread recognition of the majesty of the Yosemite region and its preservation as a National Park.

What is this disease that has afflicted so many and that has such varied courses as those of Stravinsky and Johnson and as those of Modigliani and Clark? What is this disease that has so colored the history of medicine? Before exploring the lives of some of the great pioneers of medicine whose work illumined not only tuberculosis but entire fields of biomedical science, we would do well to review the pathogenesis and natural history of tuberculosis.[6]

Pathogenesis

Tuberculosis is an infectious disease caused by *Mycobacterium tuberculosis*, the pathogen identified by Robert Koch (Chapter 5). For practical purposes, following the control of bovine tuberculosis (Chapter 1), the only currently important reservoir of infection is people sick with pulmonary disease who aerosolize virulent bacteria as droplet nuclei while coughing or speaking. Hence, transmission is airborne. It usually occurs in closed spaces with limited ventilation, and ventilation is the most important aspect of infection control in hospitals and clinics treating tuberculous patients. The organism is killed by ultraviolet light, including that of ordinary daylight.

Inhaled organisms reach the small air spaces of the lung where they nidate. They are then engulfed by macrophages, much as any other foreign particles, to be transported through the lung parenchyma via lymphatics to the regional hilar lymph nodes. If nidation occurs in the periphery of the lung, then this transport may be out to and across the surface of the lung via subpleural lymphatics. As in the case of Igor Stravinsky, tuberculous pleurisy with effusion may result. In experimental animals, it takes approximately two weeks for mycobacteria to reach the hilum. Clinically, this initial event, which is termed primary tuberculosis, is usually inapparent. In children, hilar lymph nodes may enlarge, resulting in segmental or lobar collapse or in postobstructive pneumonia. Even in children, it is rare, however, for primary tuberculosis to be recognized.

As depicted in Figure 2.1, the usual course followed by about ninety percent of persons is for primary tuberculosis to heal and remain healed throughout life. Thus it is that the tubercle bacillus can infect one-third of the earth's population, as it does today, without destroying life and civilization as we know it; *M. tuberculosis* is a successful parasite. Of those many in whom healing occurs, about five percent will at some time reactivate their infections to develop the clinical illness we know as tuberculosis and perhaps to spread it to others. There is, however, a minority of individuals, probably three to five percent, who do not heal their primary infections but progress directly to clinical tuberculosis. Age is a primary determinant of this course, with infants and young adults most likely to incur progressive postprimary tuberculosis directly. Once clinical tuberculosis develops and in the absence of treatment, as we shall see below, it may progress relentlessly as did that of Modigliani, may pursue a remitting and relapsing course as did that of Stravinsky, or may again heal and remain healed as did that of Clark.

In the earliest weeks following primary infection, the host responds to the invading organism by developing both immunity to it and hypersensitivity to its antigens. With immunologic memory established in T lymphocytes, macrophages transform into histiocytes and giant cells to form granulomas. These granulomas entrap the organisms and effectively close lymphatic routes to further spread. Later, these granulomas sometimes calcify, leaving the radiographically visible Ghon complex of a calcified peripheral nodule and hilar node, which, when present, is characteristic of healed primary tuberculosis. While granulomas are protective, they also are a major cause of the morbidity of tuberculosis. As they grow to outstrip their vascular supply, central necrosis leads to cavity formation. Moreover, their cells produce tumor necrosis factor-alpha (TNF-α), the cytokine primarily responsible for the wasting so prominently associated with tuberculosis and for which the Romans coined the name "consumption." Delayed cutaneous hypersensitivity develops in parallel with immunity, and we may distinguish those individuals who have become infected, whether diseased or not, because they have positive tuberculin skin tests.

Reactivation of healed primary tuberculosis may occur weeks, months, years, or decades after the initial event has passed; virulent organisms may persist intracellularly within macrophages throughout these often

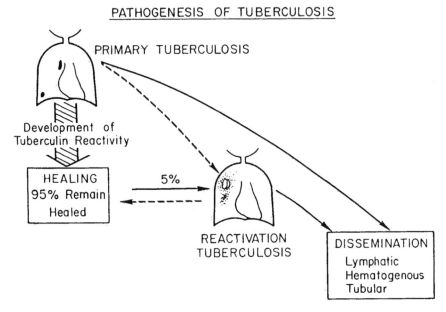

Figure 2.1. Schematic representation of the pathogenesis of tuberculosis. Primary tuberculosis usually heals, with development of cutaneous tuberculin reactivity, and once healed usually remains healed. A few individuals who have undergone healing, perhaps five percent, reactivate their disease to develop clinical tuberculosis, and this reactivation disease may also again heal. Some individuals develop postprimary tuberculosis without healing, as indicated by the broken line. The frequency of this event is largely determined by age; overall, it may be about three to five per cent. Dissemination of tubercle bacilli to distant sites may occur either during primary infection or during reactivation disease. From Daniel TM, Tripathy SP. Tuberculosis. In Warren KS, Mahmoud AAF (editors). Tropical and geographical medicine. Second edition. New York, NY: McGraw-Hill, 1989:839–51. Figure reproduced with permission.

long periods of time. Moreover, reactivated tuberculosis may again heal and again reactivate. Clinical pulmonary tuberculosis usually occurs not at the site of original infection but in the apical and posterior portions of the lungs. The pathogenic microbes reach these areas early and remain there dormantly in what are called Simon foci. How and why they choose and reach these loci is not known. Why reactivation occurs is usually not apparent to the patient or physician. Suppression of immune responses, whether due to such viral diseases as measles or AIDS, chemotherapy for cancer, adrenocortical steroids, such malignancies as Hodgkin's disease, or other causes, predisposes to reactivation of tuberculosis. Older age, malnutrition, and psychological depression all are known to foster reactivation. None of these factors, however, explained Stravinsky's intermittent course, nor are they evident in the majority of patients.

Most tuberculosis is pulmonary. The symptoms of tuberculosis are both respiratory and constitutional. Cough is almost universal in individuals who have more than minimal disease, and it is not infrequently accompanied by hemoptysis. Weight loss, fever, and night sweats are the principal constitutional symptoms. When tuberculosis is extrapulmonary, as it is in about fifteen percent of patients, then the symptoms relate to the organ systems involved.

Dissemination of tubercle bacilli may occur at one of several points in the course of the infection, as depicted in Figure 2.1. If bacteria escape beyond the hilar lymph nodes into the thoracic duct and vena cava during primary tuberculosis, then hematogenous dissemination to distant sites occurs, with bone, genitourinary tract, and meninges—the locus of Modigliani's disease—being prime targets. These distant lesions may heal with granuloma formation, and remain at risk for late reactivation. The pericardium may be seeded, usually by direct extension from a mediastinal or hilar lymph node. Paravertebral thoracic lymph nodes are reached by lymphatics penetrating from the pleural space, and tuberculous spondylitis (Pott's disease) may result. Miliary tuberculosis results when showers of bacilli reach distant sites simultaneously; it is always fatal in the absence of effective chemotherapy. Dissemination also may occur when a pulmonary lesion ruptures into a pulmonary vein, and this was a frequent preterminal event in the prechemotherapy era. When widespread hematogenous disease occurs at this stage, it is a more fulminating and hectic illness than the miliary disease occurring as a sequela to primary infection. In addition to the lymphatic spread of primary tuberculosis and the hematogenous route just described, spread of tuberculosis may be tubular, especially late in the disease, from the kidney down the ureter, for example, or transbronchially to uninvolved parts of the respiratory tract. As he neared the end of his life, the virtuoso violinist, Nicolò Paganini, spread his tuberculosis to his larynx, becoming so hoarse he could not announce his own performances. In the prechemotherapy era, intestinal tuberculosis resulting from the swallowing of large numbers of bacilli in respiratory secretions was a frequent late event.

Age is an important determinant of the course of tuberculosis. Infants handle primary infection poorly, and fatal tuberculous meningitis or miliary disease is common following infection in the first year of life. During the prepubertal childhood years, the human body is relatively resistant to tuberculosis. Individuals infected at that time tend to handle the bacilli well until after puberty, at which time most of those who are destined to develop the disease usually do so. As noted above, when primary infection occurs in early adulthood, then direct progression to disease without healing is commonly the route for those who will become ill. In fact, in high prevalence areas where tuberculosis expresses itself unmodified by public health interventions, tuberculosis is primarily a disease of young adults.

Our genes determine much about our lives, and it is clear that they also influence the course of tuberculosis in the human body. As noted in Chapter 1, Max Lurie, whose own family was afflicted in four successive generations, developed families of rabbits that were susceptible or resistant to the disease. So also do some families of people seem prone to develop and die of this disease. All five of the Brontë children and all three of the Spinoza siblings succumbed to it. John Keats probably caught his tuberculosis as a child from his mother as he nursed her on her death bed. Keats's brother also died of the disease, and when it struck the poet, he became gravely ill and survived less than a year. Twin studies support the role of genetic factors, and genes have been identified that influence the course of tuberculosis.[7]

Immunity not only limits the spread of the initial tuberculous infection; it also protects against exogenous reinfection. The strength of this protection is not clear, but it certainly exists. The nineteenth-century French pediatrician B. J. A. Marfan observed that children with scrofula, like Samuel Johnson, were protected against pulmonary tuberculosis as adults. Today, we know that exogenous tuberculous reinfection sometimes occurs and results in clinical disease. It is probably much more important in areas of high tuberculosis prevalence than in areas where the disease is uncommon. Persons with AIDS are clearly at risk for reinfection.

Since it is readily apparent that primary infection conveys immunity, it is not surprising that efforts were made at an early date to develop a vaccine against tuberculosis. Albert Calmette and Camille Guérin set about the task at the beginning of the twentieth century and two decades later first used their attenuated live vaccine strain of *M. bovis* to protect an infant in Paris.[8] Their vaccine, B.C.G., has been used worldwide except in the United States and has been given to more individuals than any other vaccine. It is probably the safest vaccine in use today. However, its protective efficacy remains in doubt. Like a natural tuberculous infection, it results in a positive tuberculin test, a disadvantage in those countries where tuberculin testing is routinely used as a surveillance tool.

Natural History

In the modern world of miracle drugs, we tend to forget that each disease has a natural history, variable as it may be. Not everyone who contracts tuberculosis is doomed to follow Mimi to an early, if operatic, death. We have already noted that the majority of persons who become infected with tubercle bacilli never develop clinical tuberculosis. Stefan Grzybowski and Donald Enarson assembled data, which are presented in Table 2.1, showing the outcome of untreated patients, chiefly from the prechemotherapy era, in various locations in the world. David Alling and Edward Bosworth compiled data from sanatoria in New York State, and these data are also shown in Table 2.1. Whether untreated or provided with sanatorium care, the death rate among tuberculosis patients proved to be about fifty percent. Others have estimated that the median survival time from diagnosis is about two and one-half years. At least a quarter of such patients recover their health spontaneously, as did Galen Clark. And some, like Stravinsky, remain chronically or recurrently ill, perhaps to infect others in their family, as the composer probably did. It should also be noted that the data from New York State sanatoria demonstrated that the more disease present at the time of admission, the worse was the prognosis.

Today, tuberculosis can be treated and cured, provided that the diagnosis is made reasonably promptly and that the infecting organisms are

Table 2.1
Outcome of pulmonary tuberculosis in the absence of chemotherapy
with no treatment or sanatorium treatment.

Treatment Country	Duration of Observation (years)	Outcome (per cent)		
		Death	Chronic Tuberculosis	Apparent Recovery
No treatment[9]				
India	5	49	18	33
England	4	55	19	26
United States	4	66		
Sanatorium care[10]				
United States	15	48	5	47

not drug-resistant. This statement is true even in the presence of such a profound suppressor of host immunity as AIDS. Modern therapy always includes an initial intensive phase with bactericidal agents, during which multiplying bacilli are killed, and a consolidation phase of several months, during which latent or dormant persisting organisms are killed. The key to success is often compliance with pill-taking over many months, and interrupted or irregular therapy is the breeding ground for drug resistance. Drug treatment of tuberculosis has been so successful that in many parts of the world, prominently including North America, latent primary infection marked only by a positive tuberculin skin test is now an indication for chemotherapy. Such treatment prevents the development of clinical illness and infectivity.

3

The Origins and Epidemic Spread
of Tuberculosis

In Charles Dickens's 1839 novel, *Nicholas Nickleby*, Nicholas befriends a forlorn and battered youth named Smike. In the course of the story, Smike develops tuberculosis, which Dickens introduces to the reader not as tuberculosis, nor as phthisis, nor as consumption, but as the dread disease. Expressing a vision of tuberculosis common in the nineteenth century, Dickens wrote:

> There is a dread disease which so prepares its victim, as it were, for death; which so refines it of its grosser aspect, and throws around familiar looks unearthly indications of the coming change—a dread disease, in which the struggle between soul and body is so gradual, quiet, and solemn, and the result so sure, that day by day and grain by grain, the mortal part wastes and withers away, so that the spirit grows light and sanguine with its lightening load and feeling immortality at hand, deems it but a new term of mortal life—a disease in which death and life are so strangely blended, that death takes the glow and hue of life, and life the gaunt and grisly form of death—a disease which medicine never cured, wealth warded off, or poverty could boast exemption from—which sometimes moves in giant strides, and sometimes at a tardy sluggish pace, but, slow or quick, is ever sure and certain.[1]

In 1828 Lord George Gordon Byron, the famous poet, is quoted as having said upon contemplating his image in a mirror:

> "I look pale. I should like to die of a consumption."
> "Why?" he was asked.
> "Because the ladies would all say, `Look at that poor Byron.
> How interesting he looks in dying!'"[2]

In 1893 Daniel Chester French was commissioned to sculpt the statue of John Harvard that graces the Harvard Yard of the Cambridge,

Massachusetts, campus of the famous university bearing his name. There were no known portraits of Harvard, and French resolved the problem of depicting his subject as follows:

> I could only go to the Harvard Library to read what few data there are recorded about his personality. That he was "reverend, godlike, and a lover of learning" . . . was about all that could help an artist, but it is recorded that he died at the age of about thirty of consumption and that gave a clue to the sort of phisique [*sic*] that he had. It is fair to assume that his face would be delicate in modeling and sensitive in expression. . . . [3]

The nineteenth-century glamorization of tuberculosis revealed in these three quotations occurred in the face of an epidemic that killed as many as one in every four or five Europeans and North Americans. Tuberculosis struck the poor. In 1845 it killed Lucille Louvet, Henri Murger's pretty but uneducated lover and companion, whom Murger always called Mimi and upon whom he modelled Mimi, the poor seamstress in his 1846 book, *Scènes de la vie bohème*.[4] Puccini later adapted this story for his famous opera, *La Bohème*, and in the opera Mimi again died of the dread disease. Tuberculosis struck the rich. The young bride of wealthy financier J. Pierpont Morgan died of tuberculosis in 1862.[5] Possibly excepting the black death of bubonic plague and with the present epidemic of AIDS still to reach full flower, the world has never known an epidemic as enormous as that of tuberculosis. Where did this disease come from? How did it become such a plague?

Origins and Prehistory

The genus *Mycobacterium* is an ancient one. Most of its members are water or soil organisms and are not pathogenic for humans. It is probable that disease-causing tubercle bacilli evolved from such saprophytes. There is reason to believe that *M. ulcerans*, which causes cutaneous and subcutaneous ulcers of people in tropical regions, originated at least 150 million years ago on the primitive continent of Gondwanaland.[6] *M. tuberculosis* has a nucleotide diversity that is more limited and a frequency of mutation that is lower than those of most other bacteria. Based on these facts, *M. tuberculosis* has been estimated to have differentiated as a modern species between 20,400 and 15,300 years ago.[7] A number of authorities have proposed that *M. tuberculosis* evolved from *M. bovis*, the bovine organism jumping to humans and mutating to become virulent at the time of the domestication of cattle in Asia Minor about 9,000 to 7,000 years ago.[8] However, this hypothesis is difficult to support in the face of incontrovertible evidence that tuberculosis reached the Americas as a primary human pathogen before animals were separately domesticated in Asia Minor and South America.

Whenever and however pathogenic *M. tuberculosis* emerged, the disease it causes (which may also be caused by *M. bovis*) was widely dispersed in Europe in neolithic times between about 10,000 and 4,000 years ago, as evidenced by skeletal remains with typical bone disease. In fact, by those early times, the disease had become global in its distribution. It crossed the Bering land bridge to the Americas perhaps as early as 20,000 years ago and certainly no later than about 9,500 years ago when the Bering Strait opened to flood the former land bridge with icy water. There are credible descriptions of tuberculosis from India from about 2,500 years ago when a Brahmin prayer exhorted, "Oh Fever, with thy Brother Consumption, with thy Sister Cough, go to the people below."[9] Early Chinese writings that probably refer to tuberculosis date to about 4,700 years ago.[10] An illness known to early Chinese physicians as laô-ting attacked the lungs, causing wasting, cough, and hemoptysis.[11] The code of Hammurabi, written about 4,000 years ago, contains a description of "a curse, an evil disease," which some have interpreted as a description of tuberculosis.[12] There are Old Testament references to consumption in both Deuteronomy and Leviticus. These texts written about 3,000 years ago were based on many generations of oral tradition. Other less certain Biblical passages from about the same time that speak of a wasting disease, which might also represent tuberculosis, are found in Psalm 106 and in Isaiah. These references may reflect early Israelite experiences with tuberculosis.[13]

The earliest certain demonstration of prehistoric tuberculosis comes from the Nile Valley. A number of mummies from Nubia, now located in the Sudan, dating to about 5,000 years ago, demonstrate typical changes of tuberculous spondylitis.[14] Representations of Pott's disease can also be recognized in paintings and bas reliefs from about the same time. The mummy of Nesperehân, a priest of the twenty-first dynasty about 3,000 years ago was found not only to have spinal tuberculosis but a psoas abscess as well.[15] The mummy of a child also dated to about 3,000 years ago, demonstrates tuberculosis of the spine and also fibrotic lung disease and blood in the trachea.[16] Acid-fast bacilli were identified in this child's mummy. The number of early Egyptian paleopathological specimens found to evince tuberculosis and the number of representations in art of Pott's disease are sufficiently great so as to lead to the conclusion that there was a substantial epidemic of tuberculosis in this early civilization. It may have lasted as long as 2,000 years. Perhaps it was from this site that tuberculosis spread to central East Africa, where it was present at the time of the earliest contact by European explorers.[17]

Archeological, genetic, and linguistic evidence all support the universally accepted concept that the Americas were peopled by two migrations across the Bering land bridge from Asia to Alaska. The first of these lasted many millennia, ending about 20,000 years ago when the land route became covered with glacial ice. The second took place between about 12,000 and 11,000 years ago, this time ending when rising sea levels submerged the land bridge. These early migrants were hunter-gatherers who moved in small population groups; they populated the entire reach of both North and South America before 12,500 years ago, when an early community was established at Monte Verde in central Chile.[18]

In the arid regions of Peru and Chile on the western slopes of the Andes and along the South American coast sheltered from the prevailing winds by the mountainous sierra, mummification was practiced, and many such human remains have been carefully studied by paleopathologists. Beginning about 1,500 years ago and continuing until the arrival of the Spanish conquistadors about 500 years ago, there are many instances of bone and soft tissue tuberculosis, with a prevalence that seems to peak about 1,000 to 1,200 years ago.[19] Early arguments about whether the bone lesions first noted were due to tuberculosis or some other disease ended when Marvin Allison and his Peruvian colleagues identified acid-fast staining bacilli in miliary granulomas of the liver, kidney, lung, and pleura of the mummy of a Nazca culture child dating to about 1,300 years ago.[20] This child also had Pott's disease and a psoas abscess, although tubercle bacilli were not seen in these sites. Finally, Salo and his coworkers identified mycobacterial DNA in a pul-

monary lesion of a thousand-year-old Peruvian mummy.[21] Tuberculosis
was not limited to South America. Although only bones remain for
study, there are convincing examples of skeletal tuberculosis from the
southwestern United States, from the Ohio-Mississippi River Valley,
and from Ontario, with dates extending from about 1,800 years ago to
about 500 years ago.[22] Additionally there are ceramic and stone figures
depicting what is probably Pott's disease from South and Central America
and the Caribbean.[23]

There remain those who believe that precolonial tuberculosis in the
Americas was due to *M. bovis*.[24] Not only must one doubt the hypothesis that *M. tuberculosis* evolved from *M. bovis* as noted above, but it is
particularly difficult to envision *M. bovis* in the Americas prior to the
introduction of cattle to the western hemisphere by early Spanish explorers. Although *M. bovis* can infect and produce disease in other mammals, including some found in the precolonial Americas, these animals
are not primary hosts for this organism, and the demonstration of *M.
bovis* infections in them in modern times does not provide convincing
evidence that they could have served as reservoirs for transmission of
tuberculosis to early indigenous Americans.

The Most Considerable of the Diseases

Hippocrates knew tuberculosis. As noted in Chapter 1, in writing of
the epidemics that struck Athens, Hippocrates said, "Consumption was
the most considerable of the diseases which then prevailed. . . . "[25] The
word phthisis was introduced by Greeks to describe tuberculosis and
used by Hippocrates. It may have had its origins in the Greek verb to
spit. Equally possible is that it derived from the Greek word to con-
sume.[26] Both phthisis and consumption persisted as words for tuberculosis until the late eighteenth or early nineteenth century, when the work
of Laennec led to the common use of tuberculosis (Chapter 4). By whatever name it was called, tuberculosis was certainly a prevalent disease in
classical Greece. However, it appears to have subsided in Egypt by that
time, and it was not frequently mentioned in medical writings from Rome.

Throughout the Dark Ages, tuberculosis almost certainly persisted in
Europe at some low level of endemnicity. Scrofula was present, perhaps

commonly, and the royal practice of healing scrofula by touching originated with Clovis who included it in his coronation ceremony in 496. A Swiss skeleton from the seventh, eighth or early ninth century clearly demonstrates Pott's disease.[27] Saint Osmund, the nephew of William the Conqueror who became Bishop of Sarum in 1078 and was the principal builder of the Sarum cathedral, the forerunner of Salisbury, died in 1099 of a lingering wasting disease of several years' duration. His birth date and early life are unknown, but it is likely that he died relatively young, perhaps early in his fifth decade. Did he die of tuberculosis? There are insufficient data to allow one to answer that question. However, it is reasonably certain that tuberculosis took the life of Saint Francis of Assisi in 1226 in Italy. These isolated instances do not allow one to assess the prevalence of tuberculosis during those medieval times. It was probably not high.

Then disaster struck. As Europe emerged from the Dark Ages and entered its Renaissance, an extraordinary epidemic of tuberculosis swept across the continent. In 1667 the physician John Locke considered that tuberculosis caused twenty percent of deaths in London; in 1790 the tuberculosis death rate in London is estimated to have been reached 1,120/100,000/year.[28] By that time the Captain of Death had already claimed King Louis XVIII of France in 1643, and Baruch Spinoza in 1677 in Holland. Peaks of mortality were not reached in Scandinavia and Germany until the nineteenth century.[29] By then one can add Chopin, Keats, and all of the Brontës to the list of victims. In fact, it is not difficult to construct long lists of those who fell victim to tuberculosis at that time, for at its peak this disease was probably the cause of one-fifth to one-fourth of all deaths in Europe. In North America, the epidemic did not peak until late in the eighteenth century, by which time it was receding in Europe. The epidemic began in New England, where Cotton Mather watched his wife die of tuberculosis in 1702, and spread across the continent, with the greatest prevalences in larger cities. At the time of the American revolution, it caused one in four or five deaths in Boston, Philadelphia, and New York.[30] Henry David Thoreau left Boston for the woods of Walden Pond in 1837, seeking relief from his tuberculosis. Driven by his consumptive disease, William Sydney Porter headed west from his native North Carolina in 1880, and then began to write the stories he published under the pen name O. Henry.

Then the tuberculosis epidemic began to wane. Death rate data are available for England and Wales beginning at the middle of the nineteenth century. They show a steady, essentially linear decline in tuberculosis deaths during the second half of the century.[31] The decline in Poland that began during the late nineteenth century was interrupted by sharp resurgences at the time of the Russian revolution and World War I and again at the time of World War II;[32] the White Plague has often stalked the human misery of wars and famine. By recent times remembered by most contemporary readers of this book, public health experts in North America and Europe were beginning to talk about "eradication" of tuberculosis and debating at what extremely low incidence could the final victory be declared. Of course, there had been more victims—Anton Chekov in 1904, Amedeo Modigliani in 1920, Eleanor Roosevelt in 1962, and many others.

What was it, then, that led to the decline in tuberculosis? It began before any credible public health effort could have influenced it. Grigg and others have attributed this decline to natural selection; that is, to the evolution in Europe and North America of a people drawing its gene pool from the survivors of the White Plague and thus selected to be those with the greatest resistance to it.[33] Before accepting this explanation, one has to note that this hypothesis supposes the selection of resistance over a relatively few generations with a disease that has its peak age-related incidence in women after they have passed through a number of reproductive years. After a very thoughtful analysis, Thomas McKeown concluded that the decline in tuberculosis in Europe was probably due to improved nutrition.[34]

The Turning of the Tide

In the United States, case reporting of tuberculosis began on a national scale in 1953. For the following three decades, fewer and fewer cases were reported each year. Like an ebbing tide, case rates were invariably lower each year than they had been in the preceding year. Then, in 1985, the tide turned; the number of cases and the case rate leveled off. In 1986, they increased for the first time since reporting had begun. And in each ensuing year through 1992, they rose further. Not every region of North America witnessed this fearsome new spread of tuberculosis. The urban metroplex centering on New York City, South Florida, the Southwest bordering Mexico, and cities in California bore the brunt of the onslaught. Finally, in 1993, the tide turned again, and the incidence of tuberculosis began to decline at essentially the same rate as it had previously.

What happened? How and why? There were several major factors. The new epidemic of AIDS brought with it an increasing number of individuals with compromise of precisely those immune defense mechanisms—T lymphocyte and monocyte-mediated immune responses—that protect against tuberculosis. The increased susceptibility of HIV-infected persons to tuberculosis may have accounted for as much as one-third of the increase. An increase in immigration to North America from regions where tuberculosis is prevalent may have accounted for another one-third of the increase. In fact, tuberculosis in the foreign-born has been increasing as a fraction of American tuberculosis in recent years, and it now represents about forty percent of the burden. Tuberculosis has always been a problem for the destitute, and the political decision to deinstitutionalize many noncriminal but marginal persons with the concomitant increase in urban homeless populations contributed further to resurgent tuberculosis. Importantly, national neglect of tuberculosis as a public health concern, born of complacency and budget reductions to accommodate tax cuts, led to a dismantling of many important public health programs.[35] This was especially true in New York City, which hosts about ten percent of the national tuberculosis burden.

Resurgent tuberculosis is not simply an American problem; it is a global one. While case reporting is unreliable or nonexistent in much of the world, sufficient data are available to allow estimates and projections. World Health Organization program officers estimated that there were 8.8 million new cases annually in the world in 1995, and that by 2000 that number would be 10.2 million.[36] While civil disruption with its concomitant refugee problems contribute to the spread of tuberculosis, on a global basis the HIV/AIDS epidemic is the major culprit. As many as one in seven tuberculosis cases may be related to HIV infection.[37]

An especially troubling aspect of the resurgence of tuberculosis in the modern era is the emergence of drug-resistant strains of *M. tuberculosis*.

Poor or inadequate treatment regimens and interrupted therapy, whether because of patient noncompliance or deficiencies in health-care systems, are the spawning grounds of these malevolent tubercle bacilli. Once present in a community, they can and do spread, bringing their unfortunate consequences to many. A World Health Organization survey of thirty-five countries found primary microbial resistance to isoniazid, the linchpin of therapy in every country, in previously untreated patients to range from 1.5 to 31.7 percent, with the median 7.3 percent.[38] Resistance to two drugs ranged as high as 12.4 percent, with a median of 2.5 percent.

In most of the world, one can lay the blame at the feet of health-care systems that only marginally reach most of those afflicted with tuberculosis. In the United States and Europe, the problem has deeper societal roots. Data from Bellevue Hospital in New York City, one of America's most experienced tuberculosis treatment facilities, provide a microcosmic view of the problem.[39] For the two decades of the 1970s and 1980s during which isoniazid and rifampin were the cornerposts of treatment, the prevalence of drug resistance to two or more drugs crept up slowly among patients admitted to the Chest Service of Bellevue Hospital. Then, in 1991, there was an explosion of new cases, and multidrug resistance increased to sixteen percent. Demographically, the patients harboring these bacilli were unemployed men, African-American or Hispanic. Two-thirds were homeless, and a similar portion were intravenous drug users. More than half were HIV-infected. They were society's outcasts—and society's reservoir of disease.

How will it end? Rudyard Kipling wrote, "An' the end of it's sittin' and thinkin'."[40] While he had a different context for his barroom ballad words, it is appropriate to suppose that the human mind can think of further ways to deal with tuberculosis as well as other diseases that scourge the people of the earth. It will require inventive thought—thought beyond simply seeking more and different drugs for treatment. In fact, we already have an enormous amount of knowledge about this greatest human killer. The purpose of this book is to look at the origins of some of that knowledge and to look at some of the exceptional people responsible for its origins. Perhaps "sittin' and thinkin'" about those origins will help us achieve the new insights needed for further conquests.

PART 2

Six Pioneers

He thought he saw a Garden-Door
That opened with a key:
He looked again, and found it was
A Double Rule of Three.
"And all its mystery," he said,
"Is clear as day to me!"
Lewis Carroll
"He Thought He Saw . . ."

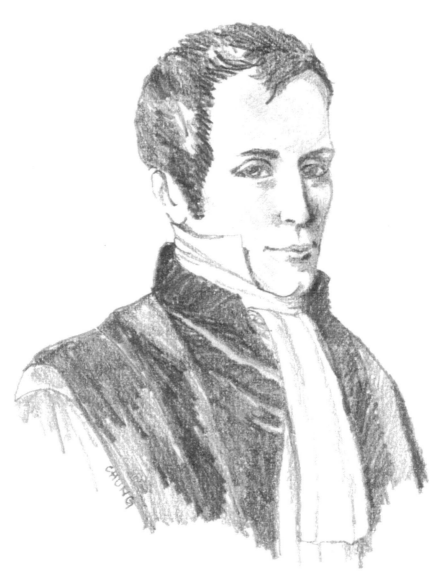

René Théophile Hyacinthe Laennec

4

René Théophile Hyacinthe Laennec
1781–1826
Pioneer of Pathology

At the end of the eighteenth and beginning of the nineteenth centuries, France was in a ferment. The radical ideas of Jean Jacques Rousseau and Denis Diderot heralded a wave of liberal thought that ultimately led to the fall of the Bourbon dynasty before the surging mobs of the French revolution. There followed Napoleon's rise from obscurity to unite France and create an empire, only to fall again with Louis XVIII ascending to the throne until Napoleon returned and again was defeated. Yet, during this time of upheaval, roads were built and cities expanded. New schools opened. Revolutionary changes followed one upon another, not only in the political arena but also in that of the human mind. Intellectual and artistic creativity blossomed. The Romantic age would soon dawn early in the nineteenth century in France with the music of Berlioz, the novels of Victor Hugo and Alexandre Dumas, and the art of Jean-Auguste-Dominique Ingres, a pupil of Jean-Louis David who was not only a popular painter of the day known for depicting ordinary people but who also fought in the French Revolution.

Medicine suffered initially during the anti-intellectual extremes of the revolution. Faculties of medicine and professional academies were abolished, but they were later reopened, and French science and medicine flourished in this post-Renaissance time. During the sixteenth century, a cadre of anatomists had emerged in Italy, among whom Andreas Vesalius of Padua was most remarkable. These physicians related diseases not to mystical causes but to demonstrable abnormalities of body organs, although they often confused cause and effect. Many of the errors made by Galen, who based his early work on animal dissections, were corrected by the Italians, who based their theories on human dissection. Then, during the eighteenth and nineteenth centuries, the principal center of anatomic knowledge shifted to France. Jean Nicolas Corvisart and his students Marie-François-Xavier Bichat, Gaspard-Laurent Bayle, and Théophile Laennec became the preeminent anatomists of their day.

Throughout Europe, similar advances in other medical fields occurred at this time of rapidly expanding knowledge. In 1628 William Harvey described the circulation of blood in his classical paper *Exercitatio anatomica de motu cordis et sanguinis*. René Descartes recognized the nervous system and its role in coordinating body functions. His work *De homine* published in 1662 is generally considered the first text of physiology. At about the same time, Thomas Sydenham wrote descriptions of a number of diseases, pioneering the concept that individual disease entities have distinct and characteristic symptomatologies and clinical courses. Anton van Leeuwenhoek, an amateur Dutch scientist who is usually given credit for inventing the microscope but probably only refined earlier instruments, described bacteria for the first time in 1684.

The rapidly expanding science of medicine began to introduce therapeutic modalities that influenced the outcome of disease. At the close of the sixteenth century the famous French surgeon Ambroise Paré abandoned cautery in the treatment of battle wounds and showed that simple aseptic dressing of wounds permitted a far more favorable outcome. While phlebotomy remained the core of most medical treatment, pharmacologic interventions were soon to appear on the medical horizon, including quinine-containing "Peruvian bark," which first reached Europe in the mid-seventeenth century, and digitalis, introduced by William Withering for the treatment of congestive heart failure in 1776. In 1796, Edward Jenner vaccinated a boy named James Phipps with scabrous material from a milk maid with cow pox and produced immunity against the dread smallpox.

By the middle of the eighteenth century, France had replaced Italy and Paris had supplanted Padua as the leading European center for the study of medicine. Among the greatest of the new wave of French physicians was René Théophile Hyacinthe Laennec, a true pioneer who carried the science of pathology to a new plane. He was an observer of tuberculosis who brought the practice of medicine to a new understanding of this disease. He related the clinical signs and symptoms of disease to organ pathology, an obvious correlation to modern health professionals but a concept that had escaped the minds of the great Italian anatomists. He was a founder of modern pathology.

Boyhood in Brittany

René Théophile Hyacinthe Laennec was born on February 17, 1781 in a substantial river-front house in the walled city of Quimper at the confluence of the Odet and Stier Rivers in Brittany.[1] His father, Théophile-Marie Laennec, was the eldest son and inheritor of the house and fortunes of the Laennec family, an old Breton family with deep Celtic roots. Educated as a lawyer and appointed to a lieutenancy in the admiralty headquarters at Quimper, the father preferred writing poetry and living the life of a socially prominent bourgeois gentleman to the mundane world of commerce and law. Laennec's paternal grandfather, Michel Laennec, had been mayor of Quimper. Little is known of Laennec's mother, Michelle Félicité Guesdon, except that she and Théophile-Marie Laennec were cousins. She bore five children in six years, of whom three survived, Théophile (the name used in his family) being the eldest. Laennec's brother Michaud, born in July 1782, became a close companion during much of Laennec's youth and student years.

Those were good times in Quimper and the Laennecs were a well-established and prosperous family. One might expect that Laennec would have had a happy and tranquil early childhood, but that was not the case. Most authorities agree that Michelle Guesdon Laennec suffered from tuberculosis, although Laennec himself in his later years doubted the diagnosis. Perhaps because of her illness, the infant Théophile Laennec was placed with a peasant wet nurse/foster mother when he was but a few days old. Laennec's mother died, possibly of tuberculosis, but more probably of puerperal sepsis or an obstetric complication, on November 15, 1786, two days after delivery of an infant girl who did not survive. Five-year-old Laennec and his younger brother Michaud came under the care of their uncle, Michel-Jean Laennec, the priest of a prosperous parish in nearby Elliant. Few details of this period of Laennec's boyhood are known; it ended after somewhat more than one year in

February 1788 when Michel-Jean Laennec left to assume a new post and returned the two boys to their father. Debt-ridden, the elder Laennec found himself unable to care for his sons, and he prevailed upon his brother Guillaume-François Laennec in Nantes to accept them into his home.

In May 1788 a sloop bearing the two Laennec boys sailed into the mouth of the Loire River to dock at Nantes. The boys were welcomed into the cheerful and loving home of their Uncle Guillaume and his wife and three children. Laennec's cousin, Mériadec, later was to study medicine and serve as assistant to the by-then famous doctor in Paris. Guillaume Laennec was a prosperous, educated, and well-traveled man with a wide range of interests. A surgeon and physician, he ultimately became rector of the university in Nantes.

Théophile Laennec entered school in Nantes at the Institution Tardivel in the fall of 1788, and in 1791 he was enrolled in the Collège d'Oratorie, where he quickly became an honors student. His education was a classical one, including religion, Latin, history, and geography. He developed an interest in poetry. He translated passages from Virgil into metered French. The rural countryside and the Loire River provided the setting for happy holiday excursions.

The tranquility of Nantes and the Laennec family was interrupted as the revolutionary Reign of Terror swept across France. Along with Lyons, Nantes became one of the principal sites of violent turmoil outside of Paris. A guillotine was erected in March 1793 near the Laennec home, claiming 48 victims during the next four months—three or four a week. Other citizens were drowned in the Loire River or simply shot; ultimately some three thousand citizens of Nantes perished. Guillaume Laennec, who had not been active politically but came under suspicion because of his prominent position at the university, was arrested and confined for six weeks at the hospital, where he continued to work as a physician. Armed troops organized into battalions or armies loyal to one faction or another roamed France, and Nantes came under siege in June. An epidemic of typhus raged. Twelve-year-old Théophile Laennec was pressed into hospital service making bandages and dressings at the Hôtel Dieu of Nantes.

Somehow through all of the turmoil of the Revolution, Théophile Laennec continued his studies, and as he did so he became increasingly inclined towards medicine. He sought advice and financial support for his studies from his father, now a judge and remarried to a woman of some wealth but still in frequent financial difficulties. His father promised money, but this promise proved to be empty. Upon the advice of his uncle, Laennec, now fourteen, began his medical studies in 1875 at the venerable and dreary Hôtel Dieu of Nantes.

Medical Studies

Laennec spent five years in the study of medicine at Nantes.[2] His courses included not only anatomy and surgery, but also natural history, Latin, Greek, chemistry, and physics. From the start, he was an exceptional student, and he often won honors and was awarded prizes. Frequent requests to his father for funds to pay for books, tuition, and living expenses went unheeded. At the same time, Laennec was entering young manhood. He studied dancing and the flute, and he sought money to buy better clothes. In 1797 he returned to Quimper to visit his father and stepmother, only to be spurned by his father who absented himself from Quimper and refused to meet him. Meanwhile, his brother, Michaud, undertook the study of law, a profession much preferred by the father and stepmother, and he was supported by his father in these studies. In November 1799 Napoleon Bonaparte became First Consul of France, ending the Republic. Young Laennec accepted a commission in Napoleon's army and joined an ambulance corps. He returned to Nantes the following March, his army experience having proved unrewarding, and resumed his medical studies.

Guillaume Laennec urged his nephew to go to Paris to continue his medical studies. Guillaume tried without success to convince his brother in Quimper, who was supporting the younger son Michaud in the study of law in Paris, to support his first-born son in his studies as well. Initially unresponsive to these entreaties, Laennec's father finally forwarded 600 francs, and the young medical student set off on foot for Paris on April 20, 1801, arriving ten days later.[3] He located his brother and shared his lodgings.

Laennec enrolled in the École de Médecine at the Hôpital Charité, which had reopened in 1794 after a five year closure born of the revolution, as a student of the distinguished physician and anatomist, Jean Nicolas Corvisart. Corvisart, most often remembered today for introducing the percussion techniques of Leopold Auenbrugger to the medical world, was a leader of French medicine in that time. He became personal physician to Napoleon and was made a baron by the emperor. One would think that the young Laennec could not have made a more propitious choice of professor and mentor. Indeed, Laennec profited greatly from this association, but as time went on he came to dislike the man, whom he characterized as "too lazy to write any book" and of a "character [that] pleases me so little that I have scarcely sought to know him better."[4]

Following the French Revolution, the science of pathology reached new heights in Paris. Autopsies were routinely performed on all persons who died in Paris hospitals, providing the opportunity for many new advances in the knowledge of disease processes. The concept emerged that diseases with recognizable anatomic features caused specific symptoms, rather than symptoms being the cause of anatomic disorders. Corvisart was the leader of a growing community of pathologists in Paris. He was joined in 1793 by Marie-François-Xavier Bichat who died eight years later, probably a victim of tuberculous meningitis. Gaspard-Laurent Bayle became Corvisart's principal assistant, and he and Laennec became close friends. In 1810 Bayle published his then-unprecedented series of 900 autopsy studies of patients with tuberculosis, classifying the various manifestations of the disease and insisting that tuberculosis did not occur in the absence of distinctive anatomic abnormalities. Bayle also suffered from tuberculosis, and in 1810 he included a description of his own illness in an account of 54 cases.[5] Bayle died in 1816, probably of tuberculosis.

Laennec thrived as a student in this atmosphere of medical scholarship and inquiry. He competed for and won prizes. His surgical skills were recognized by his teachers and his peers. Although he had not yet received his diploma, he was recognized by the medical community as a leading scholar in the nature of disease. In March 1804 he gave a lecture based on his experience with four hundred autopsies of patients with tuberculosis that marks the advent of a new era of understanding of that disease. He built upon the work of his friend and mentor, Gaspard-

Laurent Bayle, whose autopsy studies had firmly established tubercles as a hallmark of tuberculosis in all organs but who also believed that there were many types of tuberculosis—distinct and separate diseases—manifested by somewhat different pathologic lesions. Laennec, however, posited the unity of all presentations and forms of tuberculosis in whatever organ might be affected. Bayle's varied lesions simply represented different stages of the same process. He further argued that the disability of tuberculosis extended beyond impaired function of the involved organs to include the systemic symptoms now well known as manifestations of this disease. In this position he took a radical and forward-looking stance that differed from that of Bayle and others of his time. He noted that tuberculosis occurred in some persons without obvious clinical symptoms, an observation that had escaped all of his predecessors. This 1804 lecture by Laennec heralded the abandonment of the ancient Hippocratic word phthisis in favor of the more descriptive term pulmonary tuberculosis.

Laennec's student accomplishments were not limited to the field of tuberculosis. In 1802 he prepared a paper describing a series of six cases of peritonitis. It was published in the *Journal de médecine, de chirurgie et de pharmacie*, and it is today generally considered the first description of this disease entity. This article drove a wedge between Laennec and his faculty mentors Corvisart and J. J. Leroux, who wished to publish the report under their names, as the cases came from their hospital service. Laennec was angered and finally consented to a note that the cases were "collected under the eyes of" his professors.[6]

On June 11, 1804 Laennec presented his thesis entitled "Propositions on the Doctrine of Hippocrates in Regard to the Practice of Medicine." To the surprise of his colleagues, he chose not to discuss his own studies. Rather, he devoted himself to a discussion of the works of the ancient Greek, whose writings he read in the original Greek. He argued that the emphasis of Hippocrates on symptoms provided a poor basis for the classification of disease. Disease, Laennec declaimed, should be identified by pathologic features—the concept that was to make him the great pioneer of pathology he became. Following payment of his graduation fees by his uncle, Guillaume—his father had refused to continue supporting his son—Laennec was awarded his medical degree.

Physician and Professor

Laennec was admitted as an associate to the Society of the School of Medicine (originally the Royal Society of Medicine) in 1805 and began his stellar career as a professor of medicine. Short of stature, thin of face, and needing thick-lensed glasses to read, he was not an imposing figure. However, he was a prodigious worker, and he achieved increasing recognition. He became an editor of the *Journal de médecine, de chirurgie et de pharmacie*, to which he was a regular contributor. He was sought after for his clinical skills and built a prosperous practice, earning eight thousand francs in 1811 and four times that amount a year or two later. He labored over drafts of a book on pathology, which was never published. In September 1816 he was appointed to a professorial chair at the Hôpital Necker on the outskirts of Paris. He was responsible for and brought to preeminence a clinical service of one hundred beds. He focused his attention on pulmonary disease, and in his studies he clearly distinguished chronic bronchitis, bronchiectasis, lung cancer, and lung abscess from tuberculosis. All of these conditions had often been lumped under the diagnosis of phthisis. His lectures at the Hôpital Necker attracted students from all of Europe.

In September 1805, weary and in ill health from asthma, Laennec accepted the invitation of his cousin, Mme. de Pompéry, to spend a holiday with her family at Couvrelles near Soissons northeast of Paris. There he first met Jacquette Guichard, a twenty-four-year-old widow to whom he became much attracted in subsequent years, although he apparently had few romantic feelings for her initially. At Couvrelles, Laennec relaxed and recovered his health. He joined his cousins on hunting expeditions. Evening entertainments included singing, reciting verses, reading, and acting in plays; Laennec joined these activities with enthusiasm. He spent three weeks at Couvrelles, and returned there a number of times. Following the Napoleonic wars, Mme. de Pompéry moved back to her native Brittany, and Laennec continued to visit her family there. In this fashion, he continued his acquaintance with Jacquette Guichard.

Throughout his life, Laennec's relationships with his father were problematic. A spendthrift who was frequently in trouble with fiscal authorities, the senior Laennec was always ready to expend his wife's money on his own lavish life style but never willing to contribute to his son's support. At the same time, he followed his son's growing fame with interest and repeatedly sought to use Laennec's acquaintance with persons in Paris to further his own aims. Laennec's correspondence with his father, reveals both love and frustration.[7] Ultimately, Laennec and his lawyer brother, Michaud, found themselves embroiled in court battles with their father over family finances.

Laennec was a devout Catholic, attended mass regularly, and gave of himself in the care of poor consumptives at a charity clinic. With his friend Gaspard-Laurent Bayle, he joined a religious group known as the "Congrégation." When Pope Pius VII visited Paris and the Congrégation in 1804, Laennec was presented to him. This group of prominent citizens was a stronghold of royalism, and Laennec became increasingly politically active and conservative. As a youth, Laennec had welcomed the advent of Napoleon, but later, like Beethoven, he became disenchanted with him, and he wholeheartedly supported the restoration of the Bourbon monarchy. Although Laennec avoided much of the political turmoil that enveloped France during his life, he clearly had political opinions. An early liberal sympathizer with the French revolution, he was offended by its excesses. His increasingly royalist views were contrary to those of most of the academic medical community of Paris at the time. Even while establishing himself in Parisian society, Laennec did not forsake his Breton roots, and he studied his native Celtic tongue, which he had largely forgotten. When the Napoleonic wars brought many wounded Breton military conscripts to the wards of Parisian hospitals, he served them tirelessly, not only in their medical care but also as a translator and advocate.

In 1816 Laennec invented the stethoscope, a device the utility of which was immediately recognized and which brought him great fame. Leopold Auenbrugger of Vienna had described the techniques of percussion and direct auscultation of the chest for diagnosis in 1761, but his report was little noticed. In fact, although Auenbrugger's claim that percussion was his original invention is generally accepted by most modern medical historians, percussion as a general technique and especially as applied to the abdomen for the recognition of ascites, was known in Italy and recommended by Francesco Torti, who died twenty years before Auenbrugger published his description.[8] Among those who did essay the new techniques was Laennec's mentor Corvisart, and Laennec learned them from his teacher and incorporated them into his practice. There have been a number of accounts of Laennec's invention published, some fanciful and some scholarly.[9] Laennec himself wrote:

> In 1861, I was consulted by a young woman laboring under general symptoms of [a] diseased heart, and in whose case percussion and the application of the hand were of little avail on account of the great degree of fatness. [Direct auscultation] . . . being rendered impossible by the age and sex of the patient, I happened to recollect a simple and well-known fact in acoustics, and fancied, at the same time, that it might be turned to some use on the present occasion. The fact I allude to is the augmented impression of sound when conveyed through certain solid bodies, as when we hear the scratch of a pin at one end of a piece of wood, on applying our ear to the other. Immediately, on this suggestion, I rolled a quire of paper into a sort of cylinder and applied one end of it to the region of the heart and the other to my ear, and was not a little surprised and pleased, to find that I could thereby perceive the action of the heart in a manner much more clear and distinct than I had ever been able to do by the immediate application of the ear.[10]

Laennec subsequently fashioned instruments of wood, and his invention was rapidly recognized and accepted. Figure 4.1 presents Laennec's stethoscope as drawn by him. The stethoscope soon became and remains the basis for physical examination of the chest, and Laennec described many of the signs still relied upon today.

De l'Auscultation Médiate

It is unfortunate that Laennec's lectures have never been published, although most of them have been preserved in manuscript form. Jacalyn Duffin, Laennec's biographer who read all of the surviving lecture notes, discusses the failure of Mériadec Laennec, to whom Théophile Laennec entrusted his papers, to complete the task of editing and publishing them. She notes Laennec was often caustic in his comments about his peers and that the lectures contained much material derogatory of those who had ascended to positions of power in Paris. Mériadec may have

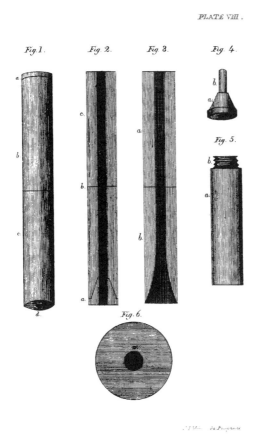

Figure 4.1. Laennec's drawing of his stethoscope as published as Plate VIII in his book, "De l'auscultation médiate." Laennec's original legend read:

Fig 1. The Stethoscope, or Cylinder, reduced to one-third its actual dimensions: a. The Stopper; b. The lower end; c. The upper half; d. The auricular or upper extremity.   Fig. 2. Longitudinal section of the same: a. The stopper; b. Point of union of the two parts; c. The upper half.   Fig. 3. The same section, with the stopper removed.   Fig. 4. The stopper: a. The body of it, formed of the same wood as the rest of the instrument; b. Small brass tube traversing the stopper, for fixing it in the tube of the stethoscope.   Fig 5. Upper half of the stethoscope: a. Body of it; b. Screw (in the wood) for fixing the two portions together.   Fig. 6. Actual diameter of the stethoscope: a. Diameter of the canal of the stethoscope.

N.B. Any turner will be able to make the instrument from the above description.[11]

Laennec turned his own instruments using a lathe set up in his Paris apartment.

felt that publishing them would not have rendered a service to his cousin.[12] For whatever reason, modern readers interested in the work of Laennec must rely principally upon his famous book, *De l'auscultation médiate*. Originally published in 1819, it was quickly recognized as an important work. It came to the attention of James Clark, perhaps the most influential British medical authority of that era,[13] who encouraged his colleague John Forbes to render it into English. In 1821 Forbes produced a version published under the title of *A Treatise on the Disease of the Chest*.[14] While faithfully preserving much of Laennec's text, Forbes rearranged it into what seemed to him a more logical order and eliminated about half of it. In Forbes's words from his Translator's Preface:

> I have taken the liberty, in the translation, of rearranging the work throughout—separating, almost entirely, the pathology from the diagnosis, and arranging the various diseases under the head of the affected organ. Thus, instead of having, as in the original, the diseases marshalled under four heads . . . we have, in the first place, an entire separation of the descriptive from the diagnostic parts; and, secondly, a subdivision of each of these according to the respective localities of the diseases. . . .[15]

While Forbes's rendition produced a work that is logically organized, it obscured Laennec's important emphasis on the correlations between the physical signs of illness and the underlying pathology. A more precise English translation of Laennec's work, which retained its original organization but again was abbreviated, was published by William Hale-White in 1923.[16]

Although the first edition of his work sold poorly, Laennec was not discouraged, and two years following the original publication, Laennec prepared a second edition of his work. He not only revised but extensively rewrote and expanded his text. He changed the title to *Traité de l'auscultation médiate et des maladies des poumons et du coeur*. This edition was well received; ultimately the first two editions sold a remarkable 35,000 copies. Posthumous editions were published in 1831 and 1837. They were edited by his cousin and professional colleague, Mériadec, whose reluctance to accept some of Laennec's outspoken comments delayed their release.

Laennec's elegant descriptions of the lesions of pulmonary tuberculosis begins:

The tubercles develop in the form of small semitransparent granules, grey in colour, though occasionally they are entirely transparent and almost colourless. Their size varies from that of millet-seed to that of hemp-seed; when in this state they may be termed *miliary tubercles*. These granules increase in size and become yellowish and opaque, first in the centre and then progressively throughout their substance. Those nearest together unite in the course of growth and then form more or less voluminous masses, pale yellow in colour, opaque, and comparable, as regards density, with most compact kinds of cheese. . . . [17]

There is no modern text that equals this description. In fact, most modern authors focus on microscopic changes in histology and give little attention to descriptions of gross anatomic changes.

The ground-breaking concept of the unity of tuberculosis espoused by Laennec can be illustrated by the following passage in which he disputes Bayle's multipart classification and argues for the unity of tuberculosis, with differently appearing lesions representing different stages of disease evolution rather than different diseases:

M. Bayle does not appear to have been well acquainted with the various manners in which tubercles develop as above described. This is due especially to the fact that he had not sufficiently appreciated the grey, semitransparent tissue constituting tubercles in the crude stage. Several of his detailed observations . . . show, however, that he had caught some glimpse of it, but without very clearly realizing the possible connections or differences between this grey, semi-transparent matter and the yellow, opaque tubercles.

Struck, no doubt, by their special characteristics he was, on the contrary, impressed by tubercles of the miliary variety which are perfectly transparent, and which he has described by the name of *miliary granulations*. These tubercles constitute indeed a very noteworthy variety owing to their colourless transparency, almost perfectly spherical or ovoid shape, smooth glistening surface, great firmness, uniform bulk, and their innumerable numbers distributed either throughout the whole of the lung, which is often otherwise perfectly healthy, or throughout a large tract of that organ although they are never found forming groups of several together. They have the appearance of having all come into being on the selfsame day, and usually no single one of them is visibly in a more advanced state than any other.

However, M. Bayle is clearly mistaken when he regards these granulations as a species of accidental formation different from the tubercles. Particularly is he mistaken in looking upon them as a sort of cartilage, for, if his opinion had any basis in truth, we should sometimes observe them passing into the osseous state: but this has never been seen. If we scrutinize them attentively we shall be convinced, on the contrary, that they become converted into yellow, opaque tubercles: indeed, there may be observed in the centre of the less transparent a yellow opaque speck, the unmistakable sign of the beginning of this transformation. M. Bayle himself gives a remarkable instance in point.

There are also other cases in which the lungs are found filled with very small tubercles, all of much the same dimensions, but yellow, opaque, and frequently in a stage of softening already well advanced. M. Bayle furnishes us again with a very characteristic instance of this kind; and although he warns us not to confound such miliary tubercles with miliary granulations, there appears to me to be no doubt whatever that the only difference between the two is that existing between a ripe and an unripe fruit. Miliary granulations are not often elsewhere than in the lungs to be seen, simultaneously with other bulkier tubercles, at a stage so advanced that their character admits no dispute.[18]

Carrying his argument further, Laennec describes the lesions of tuberculosis present in patients dying of the disease in organs other than the lungs:

Another proof, equally strong, of what has just been advanced, is afforded by the simultaneous existence of tubercles in different organs of the same subject. In consumptive patients it is very uncommon to find the tubercles confined to the lungs: almost always they occupy the intestinal coats, at the same time, and are the cause of the ulceration and consequent diarrhoea so general in this disease. There is perhaps no organ free from the attack of tubercles, and wherein we do not, occasionally, discover them in our examination of phthisical subjects. The following are the parts in which I have met with these degenerations, and I enumerate them in the order of their frequency: the bronchial, the mediastinal, the cervical, and the mesenteric glands; the other glands throughout the body; the liver—in which they attain a large size, but come rarely to maturation; the prostate—in which they are often found completely softened, and leave, after their evacuation by the urethra, cavities of different sizes; the surface of the peritoneum and pleura, in which situations they are found small and very numerous, usually in their first stage, and occasion death by dropsy before they can reach the period of maturation; the epididymis, the vasa deferentia, the testicle, spleen, heart, uterus, the brain and cerebellum, the bodies of the cranial bones, the substance of the vertebrae or the point of union between these and the ligaments, the ribs, and, lastly, tumours of the kind usually denominated *schirrus* or *cancer*, in which the tuberculous matter is either intimately combined with, or separated in distinct patches from, the other kinds of morbid degeneration existing in these.[19]

While these comments on the relative frequency of organ involvement would stand scrutiny today, modern readers must also remember that Laennec was describing patients who died of tuberculosis, almost always after widespread dissemination as part of the terminal course.

The beauty of Laennec's work depends only in part on his recognition of tuberculosis as a single disease entity. Following in the footsteps of his mentor, Corvisart, and carrying the latter's work to new heights, he established correlations between the manifestations of disease he observed in hundreds of his patients and their autopsy findings. Laennec described most of the physical signs of the lungs demonstrable with a stethoscope and established their anatomic bases. For example, he described pectoriloquy:

When turning my attention to the comparative investigation of the reverberation of the voice in several persons, both healthy and diseased, I was struck with a most singular phenomenon. The subject who presented it was a woman about 28 years of age, labouring under a slight bilious fever, and a recent cough which had simply the characters of that of pulmonary catarrh. When holding the stethoscope applied below the middle of the right clavicle, I made the patient speak, her voice seemed to issue directly from the chest, and to pass unaltered through the central canal of the instrument. This phenomenon took place over an area not larger than a square inch. In no other part of the chest could I find anything like it. Not knowing to what this phenomenon should be attributed I examined, with reference to this point, most of the patients then in the hospital, and found it in twenty individuals. Almost all of these were sufferers from phthisis who had reached an advanced stage of the disease; in others the existence of tubercles was still doubtful, though there were reasons to fear their presence. Finally, two or three, like the young woman in whom the phenomenon was first detected, showed no other symptom of this disease, and their good condition, as well as the state of their physical powers, seemed even to put aside any fears on this head.

From that time, however, I began to suspect that the phenomenon might be owing to anfractuous cavities produced by the softening of tubercles, and known under the name of ulcers of the lungs. The existence of the same phenomenon in persons who presented no other sign of pulmonary phthisis, did not appear to me subversive of this supposition, for we often meet with tubercles of the lungs, even excavated and ulcerated, in subjects who have died of acute diseases, and in whom the phthisis has always been latent.

The majority of the patients who presented this phenomenon having died in the hospital, I was able to verify by autopsy that I had reasoned correctly. In all of them I found cavities, more or less large, caused by the softening of tuberculous matter, and communicating with bronchial tubes of various diameters.

I found that pectoriloquy (it is thus I have thought proper to designate this phenomenon) was more evident, the nearer the ulcerous cavity was to the surface of the lung, and that it was never more striking than when, the lung adhering closely to the costal pleura, the walls of the chest almost formed a portion of those of the cavity, a condition that is well known frequently to exist.

This circumstance naturally led me to suppose that pectoriloquy arises from the stronger and more delicate resonance of the voice in the situations which reflect it from a more solid and extensive surface.[20] I consequently presumed that a similar phenomenon ought to take place on applying the stethoscope to the larynx and trachea of a healthy person. My conjecture proved correct. There is a perfect identity between pectoriloquy and the voice traversing the stethoscope from the larynx; and this experiment is an excellent mode of acquiring an accurate idea of pectoriloquy when no patients are available.

Sufferers from phthisis form more than a third of the patients treated in the hospitals of Paris; many facts were soon added to those already given, and quickly enabled me to recognize varieties of this phenomenon, and the practical deductions we can draw from it and exceptional cases.[21]

Similarly, Laennec described egophony and distinguished it from pectoriloquy:

Sometimes [the voice] resounds as if conveyed by a brass tube and is accompanied by a very characteristic sort of bleating (chevrottement), which will be described hereafter under the name of *Haegophonism*. This must not be confounded with pectoriloquism properly so called.[22]

What more eloquent description could the modern physician desire?

Vanguard Pathologist

Laennec stands to this day as one of the founders of modern pathology and one of pathology's greatest students of tuberculosis. Esmond R. Long, a preeminent scientist concerned with tuberculosis in the twentieth century and a historian of pathology, wrote of Laennec in 1965, "Laennec followed the tubercle from the tiny, gray, seed-like form, through the larger conglomerate and softening mass to the cavity, proving the essential identity of these dissimilar lesions. He introduced the concept of unity in tuberculosis, identifying the tubercle as the unit."[23] That tuberculosis with a variety of manifestations in a variety of organs is, at the core, a single disease was the fundamental concept recognized by Laennec; it had escaped the minds of all his predecessors.

To understand Laennec's work, we must remember the times in which he worked. The French Revolution swirled about him, and as it toppled centuries-old systems of government and society, so it also cast aside archaic institutions of medical science. A new era of enlightened inquiry was born, and in this new era careful observation and demonstration of fact took ascendancy over pontifical words. The medical world was ready for new ideas. Laennec and his contemporary colleagues in what rapidly became the important French school of pathologists were ready to deliver them.

We must also understand that Laennec worked within certain limitations. Some of them were intellectual, imposed by a long tradition that viewed the various manifestations of tuberculosis as representing different diseases and that considered such major symptoms as hemoptysis to be causes rather than manifestations of the disease and a lack of understanding that diseases could be infectious. Some limitations were technical, for although microscopes were refined by Anton von Leeuwenhoek one hundred years before Laennec's time, their widespread use for the examination of tissues would have to wait until the decade after Laennec's death when Rudolf Virchow would use a razor to cut thin sections and inaugurate modern histology.[24] Laennec owned a microscope, but he rarely used it, preferring to work with a hand lens or his unaided eye. Thus, Laennec's studies were devoted entirely to gross dissection, making his observations all the more remarkable.

Laennec himself appears not to have totally embraced the central role of pathology in understanding the etiology of disease. The school of thought termed organicism, which related all disease to organ changes and of which Laennec could truly be considered one of several founders, did not really reach ascendancy until twenty years after his death. As noted above, he considered that he himself suffered from hypochondria, meaning not the complex of psychoneurotic symptoms that word is used to describe today but rather a debilitated state thought to have its causation in the hypochondrium—the upper abdomen—but not thought to have pathologic or anatomic correlates. Asthma (a term applied to many forms of dyspnea at that time), tetanus, diabetes, angina pectoris (a poorly defined state of chest pain in Laennec's lexicon), and many febrile illnesses were other disease entities for which Laennec did not believe organic changes existed. He and his contemporaries applied the term vitalism to this category of disease causation.[25]

When Laennec arrived in Paris at age twenty, he put himself under the academic tutelage of Jean Nicolas Corvisart, joining the company of Marie-François-Xavier Bichat and Gaspard-Laurent Bayle. The hospitals of Paris teemed with patients dying from tuberculosis. The death rate in Paris from tuberculosis was probably 400 to 500/100,000/year. Laennec himself estimated that one-third of the hospitalized patients in Paris at that time were consumptive. Autopsies were routine for all patients in Paris hospitals, and these postmortem examinations were performed by the physicians who cared for the patients, including Laennec and his peers. What more propitious environment could be envisioned for Laennec's work?

Corvisart was a great clinician who brought to France and used in the care of his patients the physical diagnosis techniques introduced by Leopold Auenbrugger. More than that, Corvisart explored the pathological correlates of physical signs, an intellectual effort in which Laennec joined. And Laennec, building upon his observations with his newly invented stethoscope, brought clinical-pathological correlations to a high level not achieved by his predecessors.

Laennec's initial work was far-ranging in its scope. Papers on mitral-valvular disease, the anatomy of the subdeltoid bursa, peritonitis, and the capsules of the liver, kidneys, and spleen represented major contributions made while he was still a student. His lucid description of the gross anatomic changes of the liver associated with alcoholic cirrhosis led later pathologists to call the entity Laennec's cirrhosis, although his descriptions of this entity were not the first. In 1818 he reported the first antemortem diagnosis of emphysema, a feat that had now become possible with the stethoscope.

Laennec's efforts at clinical-pathological correlations were not an unbroken string of triumphs. In what biographer and historian Jacalyn Duffin called "the big mistake,"[26] he misinterpreted heart sounds and murmurs. He attributed the first heart sound to ventricular contraction and the second to atrial contraction, a remarkable notion since he must have known that William Harvey had shown two centuries earlier that auricular contraction preceded that of the ventricles. Similarly, Laennec heard murmurs and attributed them to heart valves, but did not make the anatomic correlations that he did so well for respiratory sounds. What a paradox it is that physicians would later consider the stethoscope a more accurate tool for cardiac than pulmonary diagnoses and that stethoscopes would be designed to optimize heart sounds rather than those emanating from the lungs. Future generations of medical students would listen to recordings of heart sounds and murmurs and apply their instruments to the precordium, while giving no more than cursory attention to auscultation of the lungs. Laennec may have been wrong about the heart, but he was incomparably correct about the lungs, describing essentially all of the physical signs now known to careful diagnosticians.

As Laennec's career developed, he became increasingly focused on the thoracic manifestations of disease and especially on tuberculosis. Bichat classified twelve types of tuberculosis; Bayle, Laennec's close friend, reduced the number to six on the basis of his autopsy studies of nine hundred persons. Laennec's series of four hundred autopsies convinced him of the unity of this disease. So convincing were his descriptions of the evolution of tuberculous lesions through stages that he viewed as continuous (but his predecessors had considered separate entities) that his unitarian views were accepted widely and quickly brought him fame throughout Europe. However, some in Paris were not persuaded by this young upstart—an "enfant terrible" who was intolerant of dissenting voices—and thus were sewn the seeds of Laennec's squabbles with such prominent medical contemporaries as François-Joseph-Victor Broussais and Guillaume Dupuytren.

Laennec's reputation grew quickly, aided in part by the obvious utility of his stethoscope, which was rapidly accepted as an aid to medical diagnosis. But this new tool was not at the heart of his fame. His lectures at the Hôpital Necker were brilliant expositions. Thomas Hodgkin, who was then still a medical student, studied with Laennec and brought back a stethoscope to Guy's Hospital in London where he later became a distinguished pathologist. James Clark, whose famous tuberculous patients were to include Frédéric Chopin and John Keats and who became physician to the court of Queen Victoria, was an admirer of Laennec and, as we have seen, was influential in securing translation of his work into English.[27]

In the decades following Laennec's early death, his reputation continued to grow. His passing did not evoke the eulogies in the French medical press that might have been expected, probably both because of his relative youth and because of his royalist political views, which were not embraced by most of the academic medical establishment of Paris. However, his reputation in France and across all of Europe as a preeminent pathologist was firmly established by the middle of the nineteenth century.[28] The great English physician, Thomas Addison, wrote of Laennec in 1846:

> Were I to affirm that Laennec contributed more towards the advancement of the medical art than any other single individual, either of ancient or of modern times, I should probably be advancing a proposition which, in the estimation of many, is neither extravagant nor unjust. His work, "De l'auscultation médiate," will ever remain a monument of genius, industry, modesty, and truth. It is a work, in perusing which, every succeeding page only tends to increase our admiration of the man, to captivate our attention, and to command our confidence. We are never permitted for a moment to imagine that we are reviewing, for the first time the mere professions of an ingenious speculator or plausible theorist: we are led insensibly to the bedside of his patients; we are startled by

the originality of his system; we can hardly persuade ourselves that any means so simple can accomplish so much, can overcome and reduce to order the chaotic confusion of thoracic pathology; and hesitate not, in the end, to acknowledge our unqualified wonder at the triumphant confirmation of all he professed to accomplish. If to anyone this should appear the language rather of exaggeration and enthusiasm than of sober judgment, let him, as a matter of justice to Laennec, endeavor to ascertain the actual state of our knowledge on the subject previous to the time of that distinguished man; let him consult the work of Cullen, the standard work of that day; let him divest himself for the moment, if he can, of all that he has learned directly or indirectly from the labors of Laennec; let him lay aside what he may now regard as the mere alphabet of thoracic disease. I say, let him do this, and he will, I doubt not, be amazed to find that of this very alphabet Laennec was the original and undisputed author.[29]

Return to Brittany

Despite growing recognition, Laennec was not happy in Paris. He was frequently ill; he imported bottles of air from Brittany and opened them in his apartment, but they did not help his asthma.[30] He developed acrimonious relationships with many of the leading medical figures of Paris, whom he considered his competitors; Guillaume Dupuytren and François-Joseph-Victor Broussais, initially his teachers and collaborators, became rivals whom he held in contempt. Sad at heart and bitter of spirit, Laennec left Paris in August 1818 to return to his native Brittany. He revisited Paris that winter, staying only long enough to see to the publication of his book, *De l'auscultation médiate*, which appeared the following spring. There then followed two years in Brittany, during which he lived as a country gentleman, seeing to the restoration of Kerlouarnec (place of foxes), the estate of his grandfather, which overlooked the sea at Ploaré on the north coast of the Breton peninsula. In 1822, two decades after their initial meeting, he invited Jacquette Guichard to take charge of his country home. She was also in ill health, although she was to outlive him by two decades. The couple were soon deeply in love and were married two years later. Jacquette became pregnant, to their mutual joy, but miscarried.[31]

Paris and Fame

In November 1821 Laennec returned to Paris, his health recovered and in need of the money he could earn there. Success and fame greeted him. Prosperous patients, including the Princess of the Two Sicilies, the Duchess of Berry, Cardinal Fesch, and M. and Mme. Châteaubriand, sought him out for medical care. Mme. Châteaubriand had been given a diagnosis of tuberculosis after a large hemoptysis. On the basis of his physical examination, Laennec disputed this opinion and made a diagnosis of bronchiectasis. Her hemoptysis ceased, and she lived to be seventy-five years old, justifying Laennec's opinion. Laennec was now the favorite medical consultant not only of poor immigrants from Brittany but of the royal court.

The year after his return to Paris, Laennec was elected to full membership in the Academy of Medicine and named Professor and Royal Lecturer at the Collège de France, a distinguished chair founded in 1542 and later occupied by many notables, including Claude Bernard. This rise to prominence was at least in part mediated by political intrigue. In 1822 the Faculty of Medicine was subjected to a drastic purge. Many professors lost their chairs, and Laennec emerged from the reorganization, which he in large part orchestrated, with his coveted appointment. Yet his qualifications for the post cannot be denied. In 1824 he was made a Chevalier of the Legion of Honor of France and also received a prestigious professorial appointment at the Hôpital Charité.

Laennec's Personal Battle with Tuberculosis

Laennec was not only a great student of tuberculosis; he was, in the view of most but not all historians, its victim.[32] His battle with tuberculosis shaped much of his short life. Although details are not known, it is probable that Laennec's mother had tuberculosis, and she may have died of this disease. Laennec's brother Michaud was also a victim of tuberculosis in 1810, but his younger sister was spared. Michel-Jean Laennec, the cleric uncle with whom the two boys lived for one year was a consumptive, ultimately dying of tuberculosis. It seems likely that Laennec was infected with *Mycobacterium tuberculosis* at an early age, and either his mother or his uncle was probably the source. Later, Laennec's mentor and close friend, Gaspard-Laurent Bayle, was to fall before the Captain of Death. Laennec's time was, to be sure, one of enormous tuberculosis prevalence in France, with all of Europe reaching disease levels never since seen in any but isolated populations; the incidence almost certainly exceeded 1,000/100,000/year and as many as one-fourth of all deaths in Paris in Laennec's time may have been due to tuberculosis. Laennec himself estimated that one-third of patients admitted to Paris hospitals were ill with tuberculosis.

As a youth, Laennec was slight of build but apparently healthy, of "frail build, small, pale and freckled with over-fine ginger hair; but he had vivacity, humor and a zest for living."[33] In 1798, while studying medicine at Nantes, Laennec suffered a febrile illness which some historians have thought might have been typhus. Others have suggested it might have been his initial clinical episode of tuberculosis, but the illness seems to have been more acute in nature than one would expect of tuberculosis. His physician uncle wrote to Laennec's father, "today, the seventh day, he is already slightly better; he keeps his head, but is very agitated, has labored respiration, burning fever, profound exhaustion; anxiety is written on his face. . . . "[34] Five years later, in 1803, while performing an autopsy on a patient with tuberculosis of the spine, Laennec cut his index finger and developed a tuberculous lesion. In what is generally considered the first description of the entity of prosector's wart, Laennec later wrote of this event, "Twenty years ago while I was examining some tuberculous vertebrae, a slip of the saw lightly grazed my finger . . . [Eight days later] there appeared a crude, yellow tubercle. I cauterized it with hydrochlorate, the scar formed promptly, and I've never been aware of the slightest consequence of this accident."[35] This episode closely parallels the later guinea pig studies of Koch, who described what has now become known as the Koch phenomenon, and provides good evidence that Laennec was infected with *M. tuberculosis* prior to the accident. It also foreshadows the work of Jeanne-Antoine Villemin who would report the transmission of tuberculosis in rabbits sixty years later. Despite the implications of Laennec's inoculation tuberculosis, which seem so obvious to a modern reader, the brilliant observer Laennec never realized that tuberculosis was an infectious disease. In 1819 he again infected his finger while performing an autopsy on a patient with empyema, but this infection was probably pyogenic rather than tuberculous.

As we have noted, Laennec was plagued during his life in Paris both by recurrent episodes of tuberculosis and by what appears to have been bronchial asthma, perhaps precipitated by the heavily polluted Paris air. He also had gout and possibly angina pectoris. He described himself as having hypochondria—vague symptoms related to the upper abdomen. It is perhaps ironic and remarkable that Laennec, who so stridently insisted that disease should be classified in terms of morbid anatomy, would ascribe some of his own symptoms to this poorly defined, "vitalistic" entity for which no pathology could be demonstrated. Laennec made frequent trips back to his native Brittany to rest and recover his health. A self-portrait sketched in 1820 shows a gaunt, almost cachectic face.

In April 1826 Laennec became ill with his final bout of tuberculosis. Plagued by diarrhea—he may have had tuberculous enteritis—he made his last trip back to Brittany. Cough, fever, night sweats, and weight loss characterized his illness. Some have suggested that he might have had infective endocarditis, but his illness lasted about four months and pursued a course quite typical of tuberculosis, which Laennec himself considered to be his diagnosis. Extraction of an abscessed tooth did not relieve his fever. Initial stethoscopic examinations by his friends and colleagues were unremarkable; later ones recognized abnormalities. He succumbed on Sunday afternoon, August 13, 1826, at the age of fifty-five. His body, which weighed less than one hundred pounds, was buried without an autopsy in a parish churchyard near Ploaré.

Hero and Pioneer

The passage of time did not diminish Laennec's reputation. Rather, time enhanced it. In 1850 the French Academy of Medicine's facilities in the Hôpital de la Charité were renovated and Laennec's name inscribed on the wall in the company of other famous French physicians. Today that room is denominated the Amphitheatre Laennec. The Faculty of Medicine honors Laennec with both a bust and a portrait in its halls. Quimper, the city of his birth, honors him with a statue in the town square.

Today, René Théophile Hyacinthe Laennec is uniformly recognized as one of the fathers of modern pathology and the progenitor of all pulmonary physicians. During his tragically short life he reshaped the science of medicine and brought dramatic new ideas to the understanding of the disease responsible for more deaths in France then and throughout the world to this day than any other. Many would follow in the path Laennec trod; few would wear shoes that could fill his footsteps.

"Life is short, and art long," states the famous aphorism of Hippocrates. In his short life, Laennec increased enormously the art of medicine. Perhaps his greatest accomplishment was a scientific approach to the art of medicine rooted in demonstrable fact and well summarized in his own words. Of his observations he said, "I hope to present them in such a manner that one cannot attach more importance to them than I do myself, and I hope that I shall never give that which I think, that which I suppose, my point of view, my theory, in a word, for that which constitutes the true science, for *that which one knows.*"[36]

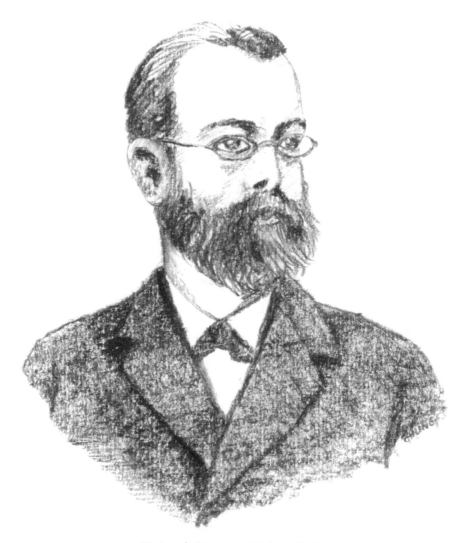

Heinrich Hermann Robert Koch

5

Heinrich Hermann Robert Koch
1843–1910
Pioneer of Bacteriology

Human history has seen a few individuals of extraordinary genius burst upon the firmament so prominently as to eclipse all others in their field. Michelangelo, Shakespeare, Mozart, and Einstein were such exceptional persons. So also was Robert Koch, who in the space of less than a decade during the late eighteenth century established in its modern form the then nascent science of bacteriology. He took the limited observations of those who preceded him, conceptualized the role of microorganisms as causative agents in disease pathogenesis, and developed the tools necessary to prove their etiologic roles in infectious diseases. He used hypothesis testing when others still relied on simple observation and conjectural theory. In the process of his studies, he established the etiologies of anthrax, tuberculosis, many common wound infections, and cholera, and he developed fundamental bacteriologic techniques still in use today. No other individual in all history contributed as much to the conquest of infectious diseases—perhaps of all human diseases—as did Robert Koch.

The nineteenth century saw Germany emerge as a European nation. Prussia became the dominant Germanic state early in the century and gradually extended its hegemony over its less powerful neighbors. Following the end of the Franco-Prussian War in 1871, the various German states were united as the German Empire under the leadership of Otto Edward Leopold von Bismarck and Kaiser Wilhelm I. Germany then occupied the territory it was to hold until it was pruned by the victorious allies after World Wars I and II, at which times much of what had been eastern Prussia, the locus of Koch's early career, became part of a reborn and then enlarged Poland.

During this time of German political and territorial expansion, a biomedical intellectual explosion occurred. Most German cities had established universities during the eighteenth century or earlier, and these institutions flourished during the nineteenth century. Medical education at these universities blossomed, and renowned clinicians attracted both patients and students from far lands. Pathology, which as we have seen had been centered in Paris during the time of Laennec, became the fiefdom of Rudolf Virchow, the esteemed and brilliant father of cellular pathology, and Virchow's pathology institute in Berlin became the incubator for the new ideas and knowledge that histologic examination and recognition of the cellular structure of tissues spawned.

At the same time, bacteria were being observed and the idea that they might be important pathogens was germinating. At the end of the seventeenth century, Anton van Leeuwenhoek ground microscope lenses so precisely that they became capable of detecting microorganisms, but his instruments permitted visualization of only the largest of bacteria. Within a few decades optics further improved, and many bacterial forms came within the ken of microscopists. Otto Frederik Müller developed the first scheme for classification of bacteria in 1773; it was improved by others, notably including Ferdinand Julius Cohn, a later mentor of Koch, who used bacterial morphology as his basis of classification. Infusions of hay in liquid nutrients were seen to yield cultures of bacteria, and microbial growth was achieved on the cut surface of potatoes. Fungi, generally larger and more easily seen than bacteria, were suggested as a cause of disease of silk worms by Agostino Bassi in 1835 and of human skin disease by Johann Lucas Schönlein in 1839.

Louis Pasteur, the French scientist and icon of microbiology, entered the world of microbes during the course of studies of the chemistry of fermentation in the 1850s, and he soon found that yeasts produced the alcohol of beer and wine. Fifteen years later he turned his attention to pébrine, a disease of silk worms that was destroying the French silk industry. He demonstrated that the cause of this disease was a microsporidian, thus providing what is generally accepted as the first conclusive documentation of a pathogenic microorganism.[1]

Although by no means widely accepted at the time of Koch and rejected by most northern European physicians, the concept of tuberculosis as an infectious disease had been born and was, in fact, embraced by Koch himself. Galen considered tuberculosis transmissible. A number of Italian writers during the middle ages thought of tuberculosis as infectious, and at the end of the seventeenth century quarantine laws for tuberculosis were enacted in Italy. In 1720 Benjamin Marten suggested that tuberculosis might be caused by "animalcula or wonderfully minute living creatures."[2] In 1868, French military surgeon Jean Antoine Villemin published a volume entitled *Études sur la tuberculose* reporting experiments that clearly demonstrated the infectious nature of tuberculosis.

> March 6, 1865, we took two rabbits about three weeks old, very heathy. . . . In one of these rabbits, we introduced into a little subcutaneous wound behind each ear, two small fragments of tubercle and a small amount of purulent liquid from a tuberculous cavity, removed from the lung and the intestine of a consumptive, who had been dead twenty-three hours.
>
> June 20th, that is, at the end of three months and fourteen days, there was no appreciable change in the health of the animal, [and so] we sacrificed it and noted the following:
>
> The lungs are full of large tubercular masses, formed, in an obvious manner, from the agglomeration of numerous granulations. . . . The other rabbit, who had shared the same conditions of life with the inoculated rabbit . . . did not show a single tubercle.[3]

Koch knew of Villemin's experiments and cited them in presenting his own studies. Had Villemin chosen to inoculate a guinea pig, Koch's preferred experimental animal, rather than a rabbit, he would have observed a more malignant course of disease in the infected animal.

Thus it was that Robert Koch entered the arena of infectious diseases at a time when all of the necessary antecedents—including both intellectual ferment and growing knowledge of bacteria—for his great discoveries were in place. The fruit was as ripe as a red coffee bean. It needed someone to pluck it. But coffee beans cannot be immediately brewed into a beverage, and it was Koch who took the many necessary steps to harvest and process the new knowledge of disease etiology. In the perceptive words of Elie Metchnikoff, the eminent Russian scientist who is best known for having described phagocytosis by macrophages and who was Koch's contemporary:

> Theoretical and clinical medicine at the time were, above all, occupied with the symptoms of disease, with diagnostic methods and the morbid

changes in the organs. . . . Hygiene and prophylaxis were in a rudimentary state. Only *antivariolic* (small pox) vaccination, worked out by Jenner at the end of the 18th and the beginning of the 19th Centuries, show[n] like a luminous object in the darkness all around. . . . At the period in question, it was the German scientist Virchow who wielded the preponderant influence; his theories of pathology became the guide to a generation of physicians. . . . His conclusion was that the essence of a disease consists in the abnormal activity of the cells of the organism. According to him it was sufficient for these cells to have developed in an unfavorable place or time to bring about a break in the equilibrium of health. The slightest fault in the cellular function could give rise to a lesser or graver disease. To give his theory as general an expression as possible Virchow summed it up as follows: "All diseases may in the final analysis be reduced to passive or active lesions of a greater or lesser number of vital elements or cells, whose capacity is modified in accordance with their molecular composition; in other words they are dependent on the physical and chemical modification of their contents."[4]

Rudolf Virchow, the most respected professor in the contemporaneous European medical pantheon, had failed to comprehend the mounting evidence that microbes caused disease. Robert Koch, a rural doctor of extraordinary genius, would unseat Virchow and vault microbes into the hostile van of the horde of human pathogens.

A Boy Who Examined Moss and Lichen with a Magnifying Glass

Heinrich Hermann Robert Koch was born on December 11, 1843, in the mining village of Clausthal, in the Harz Mountains of the Kingdom of Hanover, later to become part of Germany.[5] Robert—neither he nor his family ever used all of his given names—was the third of eleven surviving children of Hermann and Mathilde Juliette Biewend Koch (two additional children died in infancy). Hermann Koch worked in a mine. He was intelligent and industrious, and he earned promotions to rise to become the supervisor of the mine, but he was often not at home. Initially, Mathilde struggled to make ends meet, but Hermann's promotions brought increased income, and the family came to live comfortably, if not affluently. In 1855 Hermann Koch was able to purchase the large and rambling house that his father had been forced to sell when in financial straits. The ménage grew to include not only the nine sons and two daughters but two aunts, a cousin, and three servants. Although Robert was a favorite of his mother, she and Hermann devoted little attention to the young boy. An uncle, Eduard Biewend, took the youngster under his wing, encouraged a growing interest in nature and the collection of insects, and taught him the elements of photography, his own hobby. Koch enjoyed the wooded mountains surrounding the town, and mountain hikes would remain an important form of relaxation for him throughout his life. Years later, in a letter, one of his brothers commented on his love of nature, "While we gave our time to youthful games, Robert gave his to nature study and his favorite occupation was to examine moss and lichen with the magnifying glass and to study all kinds of animals."[6]

Robert Koch was a precocious child, learning to read by age five. He was musically inclined, and he learned to play both the piano and the zither. The primary schooling available in his village was limited, and Robert finished the curriculum and entered the local gymnasium at age eight for his secondary school education. He did reasonably but not exceptionally well as a student, better in mathematics than in languages. He became the school chess champion.

As Koch finished his gymnasium schooling and faced the adult world, he seemed indecisive. Two older brothers had emigrated to America, and that possibility was raised to the young man by his father. His mother opposed it, and Robert had become enamored of Emmy Fraatz, a young woman he would later marry; he did not want to leave her. His father suggested that he learn the business of manufacturing shoes, but Robert Koch, with some encouragement from his teachers, decided to study medicine, with the idea of perhaps becoming a naval surgeon. Somehow, funds were found in the Koch family budget, and he entered the university at Göttingen. He was nineteen years old.

Koch plunged into his studies. He was stimulated by the university's exceptional science faculty; later in an address to the Royal Prussian Academy of Sciences, he reflected that Georg Meissner and Jacob Henle aroused his interest in experimentation. Under the tutelage of Wilhelm Krause he carried out studies of the innervation of the uterus, for which he won a prize. Under Meissner he undertook studies of the metabolism of succinic acid, using himself as an experimental subject, again winning a prize. Both of these studies were published in scientific journals, and Koch used the succinic acid paper as the thesis required for his degree.

In January 1866 the twenty-three-year-old Koch received his medical degree *eximia cum laude*, but he entered the life of a physician with little sense of direction and no apparent intention of pursuing laboratory research, which dominated his later life. He traveled to Berlin where he attended a series of lectures by Rudolf Virchow and studied for the licensing examination, which he passed in March. He took a position as an assistant at a hospital in Hamburg, and he continued to entertain the idea of becoming a ship's doctor. Love intervened, however, and he became engaged to Emmy Fraatz. She objected to Koch's nautical wanderlust, and the prospect of marriage made the young doctor realize that he would need an income greater than that provided by his hospital appointment in Hamburg. He obtained a part-time position as staff physician at an institution for retarded children in Langenhagen, and he opened a private practice in that community of 3,000. Emmy and Robert were married on July 16, 1867, in Clausthal, and they moved into the upper floor of a house in Langenhagen. Koch's practice grew, and the young couple were happy. However, after about two years the pediatric institution at which he worked was forced by a budgetary shortfall to restructure its staff, and Koch's position was eliminated. Koch's income from his private practice was insufficient to support him and his wife. Emmy was pregnant, and she returned to live with her family in Clausthal. Robert tried unsuccessfully to practice in the towns of Braetz and Niemegk. Finally, in 1869, he managed to establish a successful practice in Rakwitz near Breslau, now Wroclaw in Poland. Here Robert, Emmy, and their ten-month-old daughter, Gertrude, found quarters in a large house. Life for Koch and his family was finally happy and fulfilling.

The Franco-Prussian war erupted in 1870, and Koch left his practice to serve as a military surgeon. But soon the town magistrate petitioned for his return to Rakwitz, for that community needed his services. Restless, he took and passed the examination to qualify as a District Medical Officer, and in April 1872 the twenty-nine-year-old physician moved to the Silesian town of Wollstein to accept such a position. That move marked a major turning point in the young physician's life.

Wollstein, Anthrax, and the Dawn of Bacteriology

Wollstein, today Polish and renamed Wolsztyn, was a community of about 4,000 inhabitants. It had been founded in the mid-sixteenth century, and had been sometimes Polish, sometimes Austrian or German, and most recently Prussian prior to the unification of Germany. Many of its citizens spoke Polish. Robert and Emmy Koch, with their daughter Trudy, lived in a spacious house with a garden and a large back room that provided space for Koch's clinic. Koch would spend eight years in Wollstein, and those years were among the happiest and most productive years of his life. He and Emmy made many friends and entered into the life of the community. He pursued a hobby of archeology, helping to excavate local prehistoric ruins; in later life during his many international travels, this interest in prehistoric artifacts persisted.

Koch's duties as District Health Officer included overseeing the local hospital, preparing death certificates, providing smallpox vaccinations, reporting epidemics, and dealing with public health problems as they were perceived. He had ample time to attend to his private patients, and his practice grew rapidly. In fact, he became the most popular doctor in the area. One of his patients was later remembered as having said of him, "What a doctor! There was something special about him. How often did I hear my mother say: 'If Dr. Koch came into your sick room, you immediately felt calm and secure.'"[7] Although he was happy as a physician, the nascent scientist in Koch began to intrude upon his practice. Part of his examining room was partitioned off with a curtain to become a laboratory. Part of Emmy's kitchen became a photographic dark room. The family budget was stretched to allow Emmy to give him a microscope for his birthday, and further instruments and supplies were purchased for the laboratory as they were needed. Koch trapped house mice for experimental animals. And he read. He obtained medical journals and studied them, making careful notes. In 1875 he traveled to Munich, Germany, and Graz, Austria, to attend medical meetings and visit research laboratories, and this trip may have provided the impetus for him to launch into his subsequent investigations.

Anthrax was a prevalent disease in the agricultural regions of Silesia surrounding Wollstein, with sheep being the principal victims but cattle and an occasional person also afflicted. Koch knew the disease, and his readings made him familiar with the work of Casimir Davaine, the French scientist who had associated bacillary rods in the blood of diseased animals with anthrax and transmitted the disease by inoculating infected blood into healthy animals. Davaine's results, while accepted by Koch, did not seem adequate to him to explain the transmission of anthrax and its relationship to apparently infectious pastures. Koch set out to elucidate the life cycle of the organism he named *Bacillus anthracis*—the name persists to the present—and to do so he developed a novel technique of hanging drop cultures. A drop of medium, with bovine ocular vitreous humor apparently the best for this purpose, was suspended from a cover slip sealed with oil over a microscope slide containing a convexity and inoculated with infectious material from an animal recently dead of anthrax. With the microscope stage warmed with an oil lamp, Koch then made observations every ten to twenty minutes.

> At first, the bacilli became somewhat thicker and apparently began to swell. Otherwise, in the first two hours, there were hardly any noticeable changes. Then they began to grow. After three or four hours they were ten to twenty times longer. . . .
>
> If one watches the free end of a filament for fifteen to twenty minutes, one can easily see its continuous elongation. . . . After ten to fifteen hours, the strongest and best developed filaments appear finely granulated, and soon small dull grains appear at regular intervals. Within a few hours, these grow into highly refractive egg-shaped spores.[8]

Koch went on to demonstrate that incubation of spores in a fresh medium led to the generation of bacilli, that spores resisted desiccation, and that they were infectious to animals. The life cycle of the anthrax bacillus was complete and the means of infection of animals with organisms long dormant as spores in pastures was obvious.

Koch's readings had made him familiar with the work of the pioneering botanist and bacteriologist Ferdinand Cohn. Cohn was a professor at Breslau, and his Institute of Plant Physiology was a major center for the study of bacteria. Koch wrote to him:

Esteemed Herr Professor:

   Stimulated by your work on bacteria published in Contributions to Biology of Plants, I have, for some time, been at work on investigations of Anthrax Contagium, as I was able to secure the necessary material. After many vain attempts, I have finally been successful in discovering the process of development of the bacillus anthracis. After many experiments, I believe to be able to state the result of these researches with sufficient certainty. Before, however, I bring this into the open, I respectfully appeal to you, esteemed Herr Professor, as the foremost authority on bacteria, to give me your judgement regarding this discovery. Unfortunately I am unable to prove this by means of preparations containing the individual stages of development, as the attempt to conserve the bacteria in the respective fluids has failed. I would, therefore, respectfully request you to permit me to show you, within the next few days, in the Botanical Institute, the essential experiments. Should you, highly esteemed Herr Professor, be willing to grant my humble request, will you kindly appoint the time when I may come to Breslau.

   With the highest esteem, Yours respectfully,

   R. KOCH, Kreisphysicus.[9]

Cohn responded promptly with an invitation to visit Breslau, and the following Sunday found Koch loading his supplies into the train to Breslau. Koch spent three days with Cohn, demonstrating his findings in convincing fashion. Word spread rapidly through the university, and the eminent Julius Cohnheim, professor of pathology, is said to have told his colleagues:

Drop everything and go at once to Koch. This man has made a splendid discovery which is all the more astonishing because Koch has had no scientific connections and has worked entirely on his own initiative and has produced something absolutely complete. There is nothing more to be done. I consider this the greatest discovery in the field of bacteriology and believe Koch will again astonish and shame us with still further discoveries.[10]

This first great work of Koch was remarkable. The scientific genius latent in the mind of Robert Koch appears to have exploded and created an extraordinary investigator out of the young doctor. Insightful hypothesis creation, inventive technology, and meticulous observation all emerged in these studies of anthrax. Seldom has such an accomplishment been equalled in medical history.

With support from Cohn and Cohnheim, Koch published his findings and embarked on the serious pursuit of infectious diseases. While in Breslau, he talked with suppliers of microscopes, and shortly after his return to Wollstein ordered a new instrument equipped for taking photomicrographs. Koch, it will be recalled, had been introduced to photography as a boy by his uncle, Eduard Biewend. Photography began with copper-plate daguerreotypy in 1839, and Léon Foucault, most often remembered for his pendulum, took the first photomicrographs using this technique. By Koch's time, glass plates had been introduced, but they still had to be individually prepared shortly before use and exposure times were long. Koch worked diligently, and in 1877 he succeeded in obtaining the first photomicrographs taken of bacteria. He sent them to Cohn, and shortly thereafter, with Cohn's support and encouragement, published them together with a detailed description of his photographic technique. Koch's pursuit of better images led him to Ernst Abbe at the Zeiss microscope company, who developed both the oil immersion lens and the substage light condenser. Koch obtained early models of both of these optical devices and described their use in his publications.

Now firmly committed to his bacteriologic research, Koch next directed his attention to pyogenic wound infections. Carl von Nägeli of Munich led a prominent school of thought that insisted that bacterial forms were not constant, "and continually lose themselves in one another."[11] When Koch read this, he was incensed, writing to Cohn, "Seldom have I read a book that has so many errors and so much nonsense in it."[12] Koch further improved microscopic study of microbes by using aniline dyes to stain preparations of bacteria, as suggested by Carl Weigert two years earlier, thus greatly enhancing their visibility. With new optics from Abbe and with stained preparations, Koch undertook a series of studies of pyogenic infections and septicemia in mice and rabbits. He described "micrococci" in these conditions;[13] later investigators would identify them as streptococci and staphylococci. In fact, Koch's observations represented the first identification of staphylococci.

Koch's fame was growing, and his friends Cohn and Cohnheim sought to bring him to Breslau. An appointment was arranged, and in 1879 Koch moved to that city. But after three months, he was unhappy and returned to Wollstein. Then, in July 1880, Koch accepted a position at the Imperial Health Office in Berlin, the city he would call home for the rest of his life. At the Health Office he was provided with a small but suitable laboratory, a civil-service salary, money for supplies and equipment, and two assistants, Georg Gaffky and Friedrich Loeffler, both of whom would go on to distinguished careers in microbiology. The laboratory was located near the Charité public hospital, assuring ready access to clinical material.

Koch was not long in getting started in Berlin, and within a year he had produced what some have called his most important discovery, the use of solid culture plates. These plates prepared on flat pieces of glass, the forerunners of familiar flat dishes which were later developed by Richard Petri, one of Koch's students, permitted bacteriologists to "pick" individual colonies of bacteria and thus readily establish pure cultures. Prior to that time Joseph Lister had introduced limiting dilution as a method of obtaining pure cultures, but that approach lacked the ease and certainty of culturing from single colonies. Koch recognized that a useful solid medium must be not only sterile but, optimally, also transparent. After first using gelatin, he later employed agar to prepare his plates, and this material is used to the present day. So fundamental is this technique that it alone might entitle Koch to claim the fatherhood of bacteriology. In 1881, Koch demonstrated his solid media in the physiological laboratory at King's College in London in conjunction with an international medical congress being held there at the time. Louis Pasteur, who had not been able to devise reliable techniques for developing pure cultures, attended the demonstration, meeting Koch there for the first time. In a remark that has been often quoted he said, "C'est un grand progrès, Monsieur!"[14]

The Captain of All These Men of Death

In 1660 John Bunyan coined the sobriquet "Captain of Death" for tuberculosis.[15] So it was in Europe and Berlin of Koch's era. A great epidemic wave of tuberculosis swept across Europe and peaked in the eighteenth and nineteenth centuries.[16] By Koch's time, it was receding in England and Wales,[17] but it appears to have peaked on the continent at just about the time Koch moved to Berlin. Koch himself called tuberculosis the most dreaded of infectious diseases and estimated that one-seventh of all deaths in Berlin were due to it;[18] in Paris it may have been closer to one-fifth. Identifying the cause of this disease was the task that Koch next set for himself and his assistants in Berlin.

Robert Koch began his studies of tuberculosis in August 1881, two weeks after he returned from his triumphal trip to London at which he demonstrated his plate culture technique. Many of the bacteriologists of the day believed that a bacterium causing tuberculosis would be found, but they had failed in their attempts to do so. Perhaps recalling the teachings of Jacob Henle, one of his professors at Göttingen, Koch set out to attack the problem with a clear concept of what he needed to do, and perhaps because of his experience with anthrax, he was uniquely qualified to do it. In his words:

> To prove that tuberculosis is caused by the invasion of bacilli, and that it is a parasitic disease primarily caused by the growth and multiplication of bacilli, it is necessary to isolate the bacilli from the body, to grow them in pure culture until they are freed from every disease product of the animal organism, and, by introducing isolated bacilli into animals, to reproduce the same morbid condition that is known to follow from inoculation with spontaneously developed tuberculous material. . . . [19]

It took Koch no more than six months to complete his studies, meet his self-imposed criteria, and be ready to present his results. Finding a venue for presentation presented some problems, however. Rudolf Virchow, who had not accepted the bacteriologic causation of disease, so dominated pathology in Berlin at the time, that Koch felt his results would not be welcomed by an audience of pathologists. Thus it was that he turned to the Berlin Physiological Society, a small organization of only thirty-six members presided over by Professor Emil du Bois-Reymond, a friend of Koch's associate, Friedrich Loeffler, and a scientist who was not a student of bacteria but rather one whose interests lay in the field of electrophysiology. On the dreary evening of March 24,

1882, Koch set up demonstrations and presented his work in a small but crowded room to an audience of perhaps one hundred.

Koch was not a polished speaker. He began his presentation slowly, acknowledging the work of Villemin in demonstrating the transmissibility of tuberculosis, citing the currently high prevalence of this disease, and pointing out that many prior attempts by others to identify a microorganism associated with it had failed. He then continued:

> The first goal of the investigation was to exhibit certain parasitic forms that were foreign to the body and that could cause the disease. This demonstration succeeded because of a certain staining process that disclosed characteristic and previously unknown bacteria in all tuberculous organs. . . .

After describing his staining techniques in detail, Koch reported:

> The bacteria made visible by this process exhibit several characteristic qualities. They are rod-shaped bacilli. They are very thin and one-fourth to one-half the diameter of a red blood corpuscle in length. Sometimes they are as long as the full diameter of an erythrocyte. . . .

Koch described identifying tubercle bacilli in material from eleven cases of miliary tuberculosis, twelve cases of tuberculous bronchitis and pneumonia and six cases of cavitary pulmonary tuberculosis, one case of meningeal tuberculoma, two cases of intestinal tuberculosis, and three cases of scrofula, as well as a number of tuberculous animals. These studies clearly justified the earlier anatomic observations of Laennec, who first brought unity to the disease characterized by tubercles (Chapter 4). Koch then stated:

> From my numerous observations, I conclude that these tubercle bacilli occur in all tuberculous disorders, and that they are distinguishable from all other microorganisms. From the simultaneous occurrence of tuberculous disorders and bacilli, one cannot conclude that they are causally related. However, the existence of such a relation is very likely given that the bacilli occur predominantly where tuberculous processes are incipient or progressing and that they disappear where the disease has come to a stand still. . . .

Up to this point my studies had established that characteristic bacilli were regularly associated with tuberculosis, and that these bacilli could be removed from tuberculous organs and isolated in pure cultures. It remained to answer the important question whether pure bacilli, when reintroduced into animal bodies, were capable of reproducing tuberculosis.

Koch next described a series of thirteen inoculation experiments on groups of animals representing ten different species.

Without exception, they all became tuberculous. Not only were nodules formed, but the number of tubercles was in proportion to the number of bacilli introduced. . . .

This proves that tuberculosis is parasitic. It remains to determine where the parasites come from and how they enter the body. This will complete the etiology of the disease.

Koch concluded his presentation by discussing the implications of his work for public health control measures.

First, whenever possible the sources of infectious material must be removed. One of these sources, and certainly the most important one, is the sputum of consumptives. . . . [20]

Others who followed Koch would carry this message forward, but Robert Koch had raised the banner of what would become one of the world's largest public health campaigns.

Koch's presentation made a dramatic impact on those who attended. The presentation ended quietly and was met by silent awe. There were no questions; none remained to be asked. Paul Ehrlich, the noted chemist who quickly improved upon Koch's staining techniques, later said, "It was in a small room of the Physiological Institute that Koch in plain and clear words proclaimed with convincing power and with the demonstration of countless preparations, and evidences of proof, the etiology of tuberculosis. Everyone who attended this meeting was astounded and I must say that evening stands in my memory as my greatest scientific experience." [21] Koch's paper detailing his work was published seventeen days later.

The passages quoted above defined Koch's criteria for proof of etiology, and they have come to be known as "Koch's postulates." Jacob

Henle and Edwin Klebs had previously articulated similar criteria, but their statements and their concepts lacked the clarity and completeness of Koch's.[22] In fact, the clearest statement of these postulates was made one year later by Koch's friend and associate, Georg Loeffler, in writing about diphtheria:

1. The organism must be shown to be constantly present in . . . diseased tissue.
2. The organism . . . must be isolated and grown in pure culture.
3. The [organism grown in] pure culture must be shown to induce the disease experimentally.[23]

The world was eager to respond to the exciting discovery of the cause of one of its greatest maladies. Kaiser Wilhelm I bestowed the Order of the Crown on Koch, and the Reichstag awarded him a prize of 100,000 marks, an amount approximately five times the salary that he would later receive annually as a professor. Word of his triumph spread quickly, largely through the medium of newspapers. Koch sent a copy of his paper to Professor John Tyndall in London, who immediately reported the results in a letter to the *London Times* that was published on April 22, 1882. Announcements in the form of cable dispatches appeared in the *New York World* and the *Philadelphia Public Ledger* on the following two days. By the end of the first week in May, both the *New York Times* and the *New York Tribune* had published complete accounts based on Tyndall's letter. On May 7 the *New York Times* lamented in an editorial the length of time it had taken for the complete text of Koch's paper to reach America, "The progress and recovery of sundry royal gouts are given the wings of lightning; a lumbering mail-coach is swift enough for the news of one of the great scientific discoveries of the age. Similarly, the gifted gentlemen who daily sift out for the American public the pith and kernel of the Old World's news leave Dr. Koch and his bacillus to chance it in the ocean mails."[24]

Koch was instantly famous throughout the world. He gave a number of talks and demonstrations to medical audiences, and two years later published a more detailed paper.[25] Scientists in Europe and North America quickly confirmed the presence of tubercle bacilli in the sputum and tissues of patients with tuberculosis. In the words of one contemporaneous observer, "The masterly work of Koch, the skill and deliberation displayed, the scientific clearness of his methods and results, certainly seem satisfactory. His results, indeed, have been confirmed on all sides."[26] Not all were convinced, however, and some continued to doubt the infectiousness of tuberculosis for several years. In New York the eminent physicians Edward Janeway, Austin Flint, T. Mitchell Prudden, and William Welch greeted Koch's discovery positively and with excitement; George Waring, New York's Commissioner of Street Cleaning, and Philadelphia pathologist Henry Formad were disbelievers.

Among those who received reports of Koch's work was Edward Livingston Trudeau. Trudeau contracted tuberculosis while a young physician in New York City, and in 1873 he retreated to the Adirondack Mountains to begin his long "cure" living "the outdoor life."[27] His health gradually improved, and in 1880 he began planning his sanatorium at Saranac Lake, which would achieve world fame as a center for the treatment of tuberculosis. He received medical journals and newspapers in his isolated corner of upstate New York, and thus learned of Koch's work. He could not read German, however, and so could not read Koch's paper. His friend, the Philadelphia publisher C. M. Lea, translated it for him, and at Christmas gave Trudeau his hand-written translation. Reflecting on that event, Trudeau wrote:

> Surely I never had a Christmas present that meant more to me than that big hand-written copy-book! I read every word of it over and over again.
> Koch's paper on "The Etiology of Tuberculosis" is certainly one of the most, if not the most, important medical papers ever written, and a model of logic in the application of the new experimental method to the study of disease. Every step was proved over and over again before the next step was taken, and the ingenuity of the new methods of staining, separating and growing the germs read like a fairy-tale to me.[28]

Trudeau went to New York to the pathology laboratory of T. Mitchell Prudden to learn Koch's culture and staining techniques. He then cultured the organism in his North Woods laboratory and embarked on an elegant set of experiments that provided convincing confirmation of Koch's results. Trudeau was a gifted experimentalist with an innate sense of experimental design. In perhaps his most famous study, he inoculated five rabbits with a culture of tubercle bacilli and kept them in a small box in a dark cellar. Five additional rabbits were similarly infected and released into the open air on an island. Finally, five control rabbits were not infected but confined to a dark cellar.[29] All ten of the inoculated rabbits developed tuberculosis; those free on the island had limited disease; those confined in the dark did not control the infection. The uninfected rabbits, although kept in a dark cellar and unhealthy because of this, did not develop tuberculosis. Environment was important, but disease only developed when tubercle bacilli were present.

Cholera—The Comma Bacillus

Robert Koch was now world-renowned, and the world was certain he could solve any medical problem. He was soon to be put to the test. Cholera raged in Egypt, and the lessons of history made it obvious to Europeans that it would soon be on their shores. France announced it would send a commission headed by Louis Pasteur to Egypt to solve the cholera problem. Immediately, the German government, not wanting to be outdone by the French, announced that it would also send a cholera commission to Egypt and that the eminent Robert Koch would lead it. Koch's only prior experience with cholera had come when he had been a hospital physician in Hamburg in 1866 at which time he had seen a number of patients with the illness. Yet he also was convinced that he could solve the problem of cholera. Within one week, Koch had recruited a team consisting of himself, Georg Gaffky and Bernhard Fischer from his laboratory, and a Dr. Treskow from the Imperial Health Office, and the team had assembled all of the equipment and supplies they needed to establish a field laboratory in Egypt. They departed on August 16, 1883, arriving in Port Said, Egypt, four days later.[30] Pasteur and his French team had arrived the previous week and already established themselves at Alexandria's leading hospital.

Koch and Pasteur had been bitter rivals for some time. It is not easy to understand why, but it is likely that Koch was the instigator of most of the unpleasant exchanges that took place between them. Perhaps national pride and animosity stemming from the Franco-Prussian War, in which Koch had served, was at the base of their strained and often hostile relationship. A lack of a common language in which they could communicate probably also contributed. After Koch's report of the life cycle of *Bacillus anthracis* and its etiologic role in anthrax, Pasteur had developed an attenuated bacillary vaccine. Initial trials with it did not go well, and Koch heaped scorn upon his French rival. Now cholera provided the opportunity for a face-off between the two rivals.

The French team, which included not only Pasteur but Émile Roux, Louis Thuillier, Isidore Strauss, and Edmond Nocard, began work promptly, dissecting cadavers and examining the intestinal tract and its content from patients who had died of cholera. However, they were unsuccessful in identifying a pathogen. Then the cholera epidemic began to wane dramatically, but not before Thuillier, then twenty-seven years old, was stricken and died of the disease. The French team was devastated. Thuillier was buried in Egypt, and the Germans attended his funeral and Koch was a pall bearer. Dispirited by failure, despondent over the loss of their colleague, and frustrated by the absence of cases of cholera for study, the French team left for home.

Meanwhile, the Germans had identified a singular organism in the intestines of cholera victims that they felt was probably the causal agent they sought. They called it the comma bacillus. However, their work was also halted by the absence of new cases. Rather than return to Germany, Koch sought permission to take his team to India. Treskow returned to Berlin, and on November 13 the others set forth for Calcutta. Such travel was not easy in 1882, and the journey down the Red Sea and across the Indian Ocean took four weeks. Once in India, it was only a matter of days before Koch succeeded in obtaining a pure culture of his comma bacillus, now known as *Vibrio cholera*, from a patient who had died ten hours before being studied. Ultimately, the organism was repeatedly isolated, but Koch and his team were unable to reproduce cholera in an experimental animal and had to settle for only a partial fulfillment of Koch's postulates for etiology.

Koch and his coworkers returned to Berlin in triumph in May 1884. Fearing that an accident might introduce the pathogen into Germany, they did not bring cultures with them. Koch presented his results together with demonstrations to the Imperial German Board of Health in Berlin. His address was published in *Deutsche medicinische Wochenschrift*, and a translation promptly published in the *British Medical Journal* together with an accompanying editorial. Koch not only described the vibrio causing cholera, but he clearly anticipated that the disease might be mediated by an exotoxin:

> These bacteria, which I have called comma-bacilli, on account of their peculiar shape, are smaller than the tubercle-bacilli. . . . The cholera-bacilli are about half, or at most two-thirds, as long as tubercle-bacilli, but are much more bulky, thicker, and slightly curved. This curve is generally not more marked than that of a comma; but sometimes it is larger, becoming semicircular. . . .
>
> In accordance with the cholera-material that I have so far examined, I think I can now assert that comma-bacilli are never found absent in cases of cholera; they are something that is specific to cholera. . . .
>
> It is certainly a strange phenomenon, that comma-bacilli confine themselves to the intestines. They do not pass into the blood, nor even into the mesenteric glands. How is it now that this bacteria-vegetation in the intestine can kill a man? In order to explain this, I call your attention to the fact that bacteria, when they grow, not only consume substances, but also produce substances of very various kinds. . . .[31]

Koch was a hero. First anthrax, then tuberculosis, and now cholera had all yielded their mysteries to the razor edge of his sharply honed mind. He stood at the pinnacle of German science, yet he did not hold a professorial appointment. His friend and advocate, Ferdinand Cohn, took the lead in campaigning for a suitable professorial post. The death of Julius Cohnheim, also one of Koch's early supporters, made the chair of pathological anatomy in Leipzig available, and it was offered to Koch. But Koch turned the position down, not wanting to leave the mecca of Berlin. The problem was solved, however, when the University of Berlin established an Institute of Hygiene in 1885 and offered its chair to Koch.[32] As an academic discipline, hygiene had come into the university world only seven years earlier when the University of Munich created the world's first Institute of Hygiene with Max von Pettenkofer as its professor. Von Pettenkofer was a skeptic about bacteria, and he is said to have drunk a culture of *V. cholera* as a demonstration of his convictions.[33]

Koch found his duties onerous, and he took them seriously. He devoted his time to building his academic department and organizing and teaching the lectures and courses expected of him. A horde of aspiring bacteriologists—many more than he could accommodate—sought training positions with him. With this, his personal research efforts dwindled, and he seemed overwhelmed. When Elie Metchnikoff visited Koch to demonstrate phagocytosis of bacteria to him in 1887, Koch initially put him off, even though the appointment with the professor had been carefully arranged in advance. The next day, Koch did look at Metchnikoff's preparations, but gave them little attention, finally remarking, "You know I'm not a specialist in microscopic anatomy. I'm a hygienist, and to me it is unimportant where the microbes are, inside or outside of the cells."[34]

The Tuberculin Fiasco

Perhaps no part of Robert Koch's life and work has received so much attention and has so often been misrepresented—both positively and negatively—as what can only be called, even nonjudgmentally, the tuberculin fiasco. Late in 1889, Koch returned to his laboratory. He clearly had hypotheses germinating in his fertile mind, and he clearly thought them important. Possibly simply trying to escape the tohu-bohu that had enveloped his institute or possibly sensing in a somewhat paranoid way that his current ideas were of special importance and might be stolen by others, he worked alone and in secret, sharing his ideas and progress with only a few close friends and colleagues.

On August 30, 1890, Koch delivered an invited address to the Tenth International Congress in Berlin. His title was innocuous: "On Bacteriological Research." What he said created a firestorm of excitement. After discussing his work and that of others in identifying many bacteria, he commented, "these results are only indirectly useful in the struggle against bacteria. We must not ignore therapeutic substances which are directly useful."[35] He then cited Pasteur's work with anthrax and rabies and surmised that ".... there must be substances useful for treating tuberculosis. . . . " He continued:

> I have tested many substances to determine what influence they may have on pure cultures of tuberculosis bacilli. Even small doses of many substances hinder the growth of bacilli. . . .

Yet all of these substances remain entirely without effect when employed within tuberculous animals.

In spite of these failures, I continued the quest and I ultimately found substances that halted the growth of tuberculosis bacilli not only in test tubes but also in animal bodies. As everyone who experiments with tuberculosis finds, investigations of the disease are very slow; mine are no exception. Thus, although I have been occupied with these attempts for nearly one year, my study of these substances is not yet complete. I can only communicate that guinea-pigs, which are known to be particularly susceptible to tuberculosis, if subjected to the operation of such substances, no longer react when injected with tuberculosis bacilli, and that in guinea-pigs in which tuberculosis has already reached an advanced stage, the disease can be completely halted without otherwise harming the body.

At this time I conclude only that it is possible to render harmless the pathogenic bacteria that are found in a living body and to do this without disadvantage to the body. Previously, this possibility had been questioned.

However the further hopes associated with these attempts may be fulfilled—it may be possible, given a bacterial infectious disease, to master the microscopic yet previously uncontrollable invaders within the human body. . . .[36]

Pandora's box had been opened. Trials with Koch's secret substance in human subjects—patients ill with tuberculosis—were undertaken immediately at the Charité Hospital in Berlin, and on November 15, 1890, Koch published a further account of his work. It was translated and published in a special edition of the *British Medical Journal* one week later. Still not completely forthcoming, Koch wrote:

It was originally my intention to complete the research, and especially to gain sufficient experience regarding the application of the remedy in practice and its production on a large scale before publishing anything on the subject. But, in spite of all precautions, too many accounts have reached the public, and that in an exaggerated and distorted form, so that it seems imperative, in order to prevent all false impressions, to give at once a review of the position of the subject at the present stage of the inquiry. . . .

As regards the origin and the preparation of the remedy I am unable to make any statement, as my research is not yet concluded; I reserve this for a future communication. The remedy is a brownish transparent liquid. . . .

Koch then noted the importance of establishing the safety of his material, and he described the effect of its injection upon himself:

> A healthy guinea-pig will bear 2 cubic centimetres and even more of the liquid injected subcutaneously without being sensibly affected. But in the case of a full-grown healthy man 0.25 cubic centimetre suffice to produce an intense effect. Calculated by body weight the 1500th part of the quantity, which has no appreciable effect on the guinea-pig, acts powerfully on the human being. The symptoms arising from an injection of 0.25 cubic centimetre I have observed after an injection made in my own upper arm. They were briefly as follows:—Three to four hours after the injection there came on pain in the limbs, fatigue, inclination to cough, difficulty in breathing, which speedily increased. In the fifth hour an unusually violent attack of ague followed, which lasted almost an hour. At the same time there was sickness, vomiting, and rise of body temperature up to 39.6°C. After twelve hours all these symptoms abated. . . .
>
> The healthy human being reacts either not at all or scarcely at all . . . when 0.01 cubic centimetre is used. The same holds good with regard to patients suffering from diseases other than tuberculosis, as repeated experiments have proved. But the case is very different when the disease is tuberculosis; the same dose of 0.01 cubic centimetre, injected subcutaneously into the tuberculous patient, caused a severe general reaction, as well as a local one. . . .

Koch then described favorable responses of lesions of lupus vulgaris, cutaneous tuberculosis, which became "brown and necrotic" following administration of tuberculin. With respect to more common forms of tuberculosis, including pulmonary disease, he stated:

> The reaction of the internal organs, especially of the lungs, is not at once apparent, unless the increased cough and expectoration of consumptive patients after the first injections be considered as pointing to a local reaction. In these cases the general reaction is dominant; nevertheless, we are justified in assuming that here, too, changes take place similar to those seen in lupus cases.

Finally, Koch noted the potential diagnostic utility of tuberculin reactions:

The symptoms of reaction above described occurred without exception in all cases where a tuberculous process was present in the organism, after a dose of 0.01 cubic centimetre, and I think I am justified in saying that the remedy will therefore in future form an indispensable *aid* to diagnosis. By its aid we shall be able to diagnose doubtful cases of phthisis. . . . [37]

An editorial in the *British Medical Journal* reacted positively but with some caution to Koch's paper and showed concern about the secrecy surrounding it:

Not even the most unimpassioned man of science can have read without a movement of enthusiasm the remarkable (and, we may hope, epoch-making) paper by Professor Robert Koch. . . .

The moment has not yet come either for detailed criticism or for complete acceptance, but no greater homage could by any possibility have been paid to the genius of a great scientific worker than that which has taken practical shape during the last week in the headlong rush to Berlin of medical men of all nations, most of them experts in the study and treatment of tuberculosis. They are all, or nearly all, actuated by a feeling of confidence in the scientific value of Koch's discovery, although little or nothing is yet known as to the real nature of the discovery itself. . . .

Already warning voices are being raised in Vienna and in Berlin in the attempt to stem the tide of misconception which is rolling in a veritable flood of consumptives to the Prussian capital. . . .

After commenting further on the importance of the discovery, the editorial concluded:

It is impossible to conclude these remarks without reference to the comments which have been made, not only in this country but also in Germany, on the delay in publication and [*sic*] the composition and mode of preparation of the remedy. . . . Dr. Koch has earned the confidence and respect of the medical profession, and our patience is not to be severely taxed, for it is much to be hoped that Dr. Koch may adhere to the arrangement which he is understood to have made, and will give at an early date the promised account of the mode of preparation of his remedy.[38]

Much has been written of the rush to Berlin—a commentator in Lancet called it an hegira—of both physicians and tuberculous patients that followed Koch's presentation. A colorful commentary in the British periodical *Review of Reviews* stated:

> Europe witnessed a strange but not unprecedented spectacle last month. In the Middle Ages the discovery of a new wonder-working shrine, or the establishment of the repute of the grave of a saint as a fount of miracles, often led to the same rush which has taken place last month to Berlin. "'Tis for life, for life ye fly!" As in Macaulay's vivid picture of the flight of the Antediluvians from the advancing waters of the flood, the consumptive patients of the Continent have been stampeding for dear life to the capital of Germany. The dying have hurried thither, sometimes to expire in the railway train, but buoyed up for a time by a new potent hope—a hope that at last the wizards of science had discovered a formula by which to conjure away the malady which has eaten its way into their lungs. It is a melancholy reflection that there will probably be more patients killed by exposure or neglect in the overcrowded lodgings of Berlin than Dr. Koch is likely to cure for many a long day to come, but no one can be surprised at the readiness of the despairing to resort to the new pool of Siloam which science seems to have opened in the capital of Germany.[39]

Sir Joseph Lister was among those who went to Berlin. He reported in a lecture at King's College Hospital on December 3, 1890:

> Having just returned from a visit of a few days to Berlin, were I have had the opportunity of witnessing Koch's treatment of tuberculosis, I will relate to you some of my impressions regarding it. . . . The effects of this treatment upon tubercular disease are simply astounding.[40]

Arthur Conan Doyle, whom many remember as the author of Sherlock Holmes stories while forgetting that he was a distinguished physician, joined the flock of Berlin-bound lemmings. His wife suffered from tuberculosis, and this, in part, may have motivated him to go. He wrote a revealing account of his experience that provides a look not only at the treatment but at Koch and his institute:

> To the Englishman in Berlin, and indeed to the German also, it is at present very much easier to see the bacillus of Koch, that to catch even the most fleeting glimpse of its illustrious discoverer. His name is on every lip, his utterances are the constant subject of conversation, but,

like the Veiled Prophet, he still remains unseen to any eyes save those of his own immediate coworkers and assistants. The stranger must content himself by looking up at the long grey walls of the Hygiene Museum in Kloster Strasse, and knowing that somewhere within them the great master mind is working, which is rapidly bringing under subjection those unruly tribes of deadly micro-organisms which are the last creatures in the organic world to submit to the sway of man. . . .

The great bacteriologist is a man so devoted to his own particular line of work that all descriptions of him from other points of view must, in the main, be negative. Some five feet and a half in height, sturdily built, with brown hair fringing off to grey at the edges, he is a man whose appearance might be commonplace were it not for the vivacity of his expression and the quick decision of his manner. Of a thoroughly German type, with his earnest face, his high thoughtful forehead, and his slightly retroussé nose, he looks what he is, a student, a worker, and a philosopher. His eyes are small, grey, and searching, but so sorely tried by long years of microscopic work that they require the aid of the strongest glasses. A married man, and of a domestic turn of mind, his life is spent either in the complete privacy of his family, or in the absorbing labour of his laboratory. He smokes little, drinks less, and leads so regular a life that he reserves his whole energy for the all-important mission to which he has devoted himself. . . .

To his own private sanctum few, as has already been remarked, can gain access, but in the Kloster Strasse there is his public laboratory, in which some fifty young men, including several Americans and Englishmen, are pursuing their studies in bacteriology. It is a large square chamber, well lit and lofty, with rows of microscopes bristling along the deal tables which line it upon every side. . . .

As to the efficacy of the treatment, the skepticism with which it has been encountered in some quarters is as undeserved as the absolute confidence with which others have hailed it. It must never be lost sight of that Koch has never claimed that his fluid kills the tubercle bacillus. On the contrary, it has no effect upon it, but destroys the low form of tissue in the meshes of which the bacilli lie. Should this tissue slough in the case of lupus, or be expelled in the sputum in the case of phthisis, and should it contain in its meshes all the bacilli, then it would be possible to hope for a complete cure. When one considers, however, the number and the minute size of these deadly organisms, and the evidence that the lymphatics as well as the organs are affected by them, it is evident that it will only be in very exceptional cases that the bacilli are all expelled. . . .

There can be no question that it forms an admirable aid to diagnosis. Tubercle, and tubercle alone, responds to its action, so that in all cases where the exact nature of a complaint is doubtful, a single injection is enough to determine whether it is scrofulous, lupous, phthisical, or in any way tuberculous. This alone is a very important addition to the art of medicine.

Lastly, as to the obtaining of the all-important lymph, I called upon Dr. A. Libbertz, to whom its distribution has been entrusted, and I learned that the present supply is insufficient to meet the demands, even of the Berlin hospitals, and that it will be months before any other applicants can be supplied. A pile of letters upon the floor, four feet across, and as high as a man's knee, gave some indication as to what the future demand would be. These, I was informed, represented a single post.[41]

The secrecy over the nature of Koch's remedy ended in January 1891, when Koch revealed that it was, in fact, the sterile, glycerine-rich supernatant of cultures of tubercle bacilli. The name tuberculin was given to it by Dr. Libbertz, the long-time friend to whom Koch had entrusted its distribution.

It was not long before a summary of treatment results achieved with Koch's tuberculin was published by a commission of the German government. The results were promptly reported in the *British Medical Journal*. They are summarized in Table 5.1. Clearly, the hoped-for miracle was more of an illusion than a reality.

Among the observations to come out of Koch's studies of tuberculin were some sound and important studies performed in guinea pigs. They are well described in his words as translated by Graham Bothamley and John Grange:

> If a healthy guinea-pig is inoculated with a pure culture of tubercle bacilli, the inoculation wound usually closes and appears to heal within a few days; however, after 10–14 days a hard nodule appears and soon breaks down to form an ulcer which remains until the animal dies. By contrast, something quite different happens when a guinea-pig already ill with tuberculosis is inoculated. . . . In such an animal the small inoculation wound also closes initially but no nodule develops; instead a peculiar change occurs at the inoculation site over the next day or two. The region becomes hard and darkened: this is not restricted to the inoculation point but spreads out to a diameter of 0.0–1.0 cm. During the

Table 5.1

Results of treatment of tuberculosis with Koch's tuberculin.
Because of incomplete reporting of cases, the numbers in the outcomes
columns do not equal the number of cases treated. Data used in this table are
drawn from the official report on the results of Koch's treatment in Prussia.[42]

	Outcomes		
Form of Disease	Number Treated	Cured	Improved	Unimproved or Died
Pulmonary Tuberculosis				
Early	242	9	131	93
Moderately advanced	444	1	136	284
Very advanced	246	0	38	192
Extrapulmonary tuberculosis				
Lupus vulgaris	188	5	162	21
All others	690	10	223	286

following few days the altered skin becomes necrotic and sloughs off, leaving a flat ulcer which usually heals rapidly and permanently without involvement of the neighboring lymph nodes. Hence, the inoculated tubercle bacilli affect the skin of a healthy animal in a quite different manner than that of a tuberculous one. This remarkable effect is not caused exclusively by living tubercle bacilli but also by killed ones. . . . [43]

To Koch, this effect, which has come to known as the Koch phenomenon, provided a rational explanation for the results of his treatment of cutaneous tuberculosis with tuberculin, and it offered hope for a bacterial vaccine against tuberculosis. To the world of succeeding generations of immunologists it provides the elegant first demonstration of what we now know to be cell-mediated immunity. It spawned understanding of immunological reactions that have importance to cancer, many infectious diseases, and many autoimmune phenomena. To readers of this book, it casts informative light on Laennec's description of his accidental tuberculous wound (Chapter 4).

Looking back from the perspective of more than a century during which much has been learned about the immunology of tuberculosis, what can be said of Koch's failed remedy? First of all, there were ample precedents for what Koch did. Jenner had shown that vaccinia prevented variola. Pasteur had shown that an attenuated rabies virus, *given after infection*, prevented rabies. Koch was giving tuberculin antigens, and it was not unreasonable for him to hypothesize that the response to them might influence the course of disease. Even today, at the start of the twenty-first century, there is a renewed interest in using avirulent *Mycobacterium vaccae* as a post-infection vaccine to stimulate the immunity of patients suffering from advanced tuberculosis with the hope of ameliorating their disease. Secondly, it should be noted that Koch approached his new therapy with some caution, establishing its safety first in animals and then in healthy volunteers, notably including himself.

Next is the issue of Koch's secrecy, an anathema in the scientific world then and now. The *Journal of the American Medical Association* defended Koch's approach as the only way to prevent charlatans from exploiting his name with spurious products.[44] In fact, this was not long in happening.

Finally, in defense of Koch, he was under considerable pressure from German government officials to produce dramatic results, and this pressure may have led him to speak out before he was fully prepared to do so.[45] However, before we further exculpate Koch, we must also note that he, and especially the clinical colleagues to whom he entrusted the clinical trials of tuberculin, stood to gain great financial benefit from this treatment that they and only they could provide. In the end, one wishes that Koch had not proposed tuberculin therapy for tuberculosis. However, when viewed against the standards of his time and even against the practices of today, it is hard to fault him. He was mistaken; he was not malintentioned.

Dénouement

Within one glorious decade, Robert Koch had found the causes of anthrax, many common wound infections, tuberculosis, and cholera. In the process, he had developed the fundamental laboratory techniques that underlie the study of bacteria to this day. He had then become embroiled in the morass of tuberculin, a substance he did not understand and that would have to await the studies of Clemens von Pirquet and subsequent generations of immunologists to unravel. The last two decades of his life saw him retreat further and further from public view. Although he continued to investigate infectious diseases, he made no further remarkable discoveries of the sort the world had come to expect of him. A new Institute for Infectious Diseases, with both clinical and laboratory facilities, was built for Koch; it opened in November 1890, just as the tuberculin maelstrom was about to engulf him. Koch was given a salary of 20,000 marks annually. While much illustrious work was done at that institute, it was not Koch's work but that of his many students and protegés that made it famous.

During the years in Berlin, Robert and Emmy Koch's marriage slowly fell apart. Despite the comments by Arthur Conan Doyle quoted above, Koch was not "of a domestic turn of mind," and he largely ignored his wife after their move to Berlin, perhaps because he was totally engrossed in his studies, more likely because they had fewer and fewer interests in common. It is remarkable that he wrote frequent letters to his beloved daughter, Trudy, from Egypt and India during his quest for *V. cholera*, but only occasionally corresponded with his wife. In 1888, Trudy married Eduard Pfuhl, one of Koch's young associates; Koch was not happy at this event, and the loss of his daughter probably contributed to his further estrangement from his wife. He is said to have become depressed, secretive, and perhaps paranoid following his daughter's marriage. The following year Koch met Hedwig Freiberg, a seventeen-year-old art student and part-time actress. Accounts of how they met differ among Koch's biographers. It is said that he saw her picture in a barber shop and sought her out. More likely, he became acquainted with her when she played a small part in a play that he saw, as he frequently attended the theater for relaxation. Hedwig Freiberg and Robert Koch were soon in love. She was not only strikingly pretty; she was intelligent and showed great interest in his work, which Emmy had not done since leaving Wollstein.

Koch had purchased and refurbished his old family home in Clausthal in 1890. In 1893 he and Emmy were divorced. As part of the settlement, she gained the Clausthal house, to which she moved and where she lived for the rest of her life. Meanwhile, Trudy and her husband Eduard Pfuhl, had moved to Strassburg. Koch was alone in Berlin, but not for long. The forty-nine-year-old Robert Koch and twenty-year-old Hedwig Freiberg were married on September 13, 1893.

The establishment of German professors was scandalized. Tongues wagged. Elie Metchnikoff recalled:

[Koch's romance] unleashed a moral storm, as was to be expected. During the Congress of German Physicians in 1892, where I was present, Koch's marriage was the topic of all conversation. Koch, whose scientific greatness had not as yet been forgiven him [*sic*], was exposed to the most serious accusations; his romance certainly interested the professors more than all the reports submitted to the Congress.[46]

Years later, the couple visited Saranac Lake and met Edward Livingston Trudeau, who is said to have commented, "You could not blame Koch, but what on earth could the young woman see in him!"[47]

Koch's marriage to the young Hedwig was enormously successful. Hedwig was devoted to him. She shared his interest in travel, was willing to tolerate the inconveniences of the journeys to remote places that fascinated Koch, and she served as his English-language translator.

In 1896 Koch escaped from Berlin, and the remainder of his life would be focused elsewhere. An epidemic of rinderpest was decimating the herds of cattle in the South African British colonies. The British Colonial Office turned to Koch, and in November, accompanied by Hedwig, he set forth for South Africa. He established a research station in Kimberly in facilities provided by the De Beers diamond-mining company. Rinderpest is a viral disease, and Koch made no progress in his attempts to isolate an etiologic bacterium. Building on work already underway by South African investigators, he found that passive immunization with serum protected animals. He then developed a successful immunization method using bile from animals that had died of the disease. The rinderpest virus is excreted in bile, and it is probable that it is attenuated sufficiently by bile salts to have served as a vaccine. With or without Koch's efforts, the rinderpest epidemic ran its course and subsided by the end of 1898.[48]

While Koch was in South Africa, an epidemic of plague erupted in India and was threatening the ports of Europe. Alexandre Yersin had demonstrated that plague was caused by a bacterium (which now is called *Yersinia pestis*) and rat-borne fleas were known to be the major vector. Koch was still an employee of the German government, and he was ordered to proceed to India to report on the epidemic. This he did, reporting back that efforts to control rats must be increased, but he stayed only a short time in India. July 1897 found him in Dar es Salaam, the principal port city of German East Africa, where he spent the next year studying malaria and trypanosomiasis, returning to Berlin in May 1889. One year later he was again traveling, this time to Indonesia, again studying malaria. In none of these internationally conducted studies did Koch do more than confirm the findings of previous workers.

Koch's reputation in Europe remained undiminished. In 1900 a new and enlarged institute was opened for him in Berlin, an institute that was ultimately to be named the Robert Koch Institute. In 1902 Rudolf Virchow died, leaving vacancies in the French and Austrian Academy of Sciences. Robert Koch was elected to fill these positions. In 1904, Koch retired from his institute directorship, being succeeded by his long-time friend and colleague, Georg Gaffky. And in that year he returned to his beloved Africa, setting up camp on the shores of Lake Victoria to study trypanosomiasis.

In 1905 Robert Koch was awarded the Nobel Prize in Medicine or Physiology, the fifth person to receive this prestigious award. He was bitter about having been passed over for the first four awards of the prize, and a review of the awardees in Table 5.2 does lead one to wonder about the judgement of the faculty members at the Carolinska Institute who voted for them. Von Behring's work was certainly important, although it must have been disappointing to Koch that his young pupil should precede him; and so also was the work of Ross important. As for the now totally forgotten work of Finsen and Pavlov's salivating dogs, one can only say that history has judged Koch's work on tuberculosis as far more important.

Koch's Nobel lecture was entitled "How the Fight against Tuberculosis Now Stands," and it was a remarkable presentation, for it concerned itself with public health rather than bacteriology. He made two major points concerning the transmission of tuberculosis, one of which appears to have reflected a departure from his usually critical thinking, and the other of which was remarkably prescient. The first concerned bovine tuberculosis:

> [W]e must attain to absolute clearness as to the manner in which infection in tuberculosis takes place—i.e., as to how the tubercle bacilli get

Table 5.2
Winners of the Nobel Prize in Medicine or Physiology, 1901 through 1905.

1901	Emil von Behring	Treatment of diphtheria with immune serum.
1902	Ronald Ross	Identification of the life cycle of the malaria parasite and its transmission by mosquitos.
1903	Niels Ryberg Finsen	Light therapy of skin diseases.
1904	Ivan Petrovich Pavlov	Studies on the physiology of digestion.
1905	Robert Koch	Discovery of the etiology of tuberculosis.

into the human organism, for the sole purpose of all prophylactic measures against a pestilence must be to prevent the entrance of the germs of
disease into man. Now, as regards infection with tuberculosis only two
possibilities have hitherto presented themselves—namely, infection by
tubercle bacilli emanating from tuberculous human beings and infection by tubercle bacilli contained in the flesh and milk of tuberculous
cattle. After the investigations which I have made. . . . we may dismiss
this second possibility, or at least regard it as so slight that this source of
infection as compared with the other falls quite into the background.
We arrived, namely, at the result that human tuberculosis and bovine
tuberculosis are different from one another and that bovine tuberculosis
is not transmissible to man.[49]

The idea that bovine tuberculosis was different from the human form
and did not present a public health threat was first espoused by Koch at
the International Congress on Tuberculosis of London in 1901, and it
represented a reversal of his previous position on this subject. At that
meeting Koch presented the results of his unsuccessful attempt to infect
cattle with organisms isolated from humans. However, his experiments
were not confirmed by others, and evidence for bovine infection of
humans was mounting day by day.[50]

Koch then turned to human transmission of tuberculosis:

But now the disease does not in all cases assume such forms that tubercle
bacilli are expelled in a manner deserving of attention. Strictly speaking,
it is only those who suffer from laryngeal and pulmonary tuberculosis
that produce considerable quantities of tubercle bacilli and disseminate
them in a dangerous manner. At the same time, however, attention must
be paid to the fact that it is not only the secretion of the lungs called sputum

that is dangerous as containing bacilli, but that according to Flügge's investigations the minutest droplets of phlegm that are flung into the air by the patients when they cough and clear their throats and even when they speak also contain bacilli and can thereby cause infection. . . .

For the healthy the danger of infection increases with the impossibility of avoiding the immediate neighborhood of a dangerous patient— i.e., in densely inhabited rooms, and quite specially if the latter are not only overcrowded but also badly ventilated and inadequately lighted.

I now address myself to the task of testing the measures now in force as to the degree in which they take the etiological facts just stated into account. . . .

The starting-point for the combating of all pestilences is *notification*, because without it most cases of disease would remain unknown. So we must demand it for tuberculosis too. But in the case of this disease the competent parties have, out of consideration for the patients, scrupled to prescribe notification to the medical men or those on whom the obligation lies in other cases.[51]

As we will observe in Chapter 6, Koch had been in contact with Hermann Biggs, who had instituted reporting of tuberculosis in New York, and Koch much admired his efforts. Koch then concluded his remarks by calling for isolation of infectious cases. Clearly Koch was again ready to exert leadership within his profession, this time not with microscope and culture plate but with public health regulations.

Scarcely had Koch returned from accepting the Nobel Prize in Stockholm when he set out for Africa again to continue his studies of trypanosomiasis. Hedwig again went with him, but soon had to return after she became ill with malaria. Koch stayed in East Africa for eighteen months.

In 1908 Robert and Hedwig Koch again journeyed forth, this time with the intention of circling the globe. They sailed to New York, where Koch met with Hermann Biggs and others in the health department he much admired. They then visited Koch's two brothers in the midwest before continuing across the continent to San Francisco and embarking for Japan, where they were hosted by Koch's former student Shibasaburo Kitasato, now Director of the Institute for Infectious Diseases of Tokyo.

In Tokyo the Kochs' grand tour was interrupted by an urgent request to reverse his travel and attend the Sixth International Conference on

Tuberculosis to be held at the Willard Hotel in Washington. The American bacteriologist Theobald Smith had proclaimed the bovine tubercle bacillus a distinct species and he insisted on its infectiousness to humans. Koch was urged to attend to present the German view, which he did, adamantly adhering to the position he had stated seven years earlier in his Nobel lecture. As the conference moved closer to issuing a formal consensus statement, it also became more fractious. Hermann Biggs stepped in to mediate. Ultimately, Koch yielded, although continuing to insist that bovine tuberculosis was a relatively unimportant public health problem.[52] And, at the close of this conference, the sweeping campaign that led to the eradication of bovine tuberculosis in North America was launched. Its dramatic success is recounted in Chapter 1.

Koch returned from Washington to Berlin, and his health began to fail. In a letter to his daughter, Trudy, written in December 1903, he had referred to "little indications that everything inside might not be completely all right: heart pains, shortness of breath, but the symptoms don't last."[53]

One can now recognize these symptoms as angina pectoris and perhaps heart failure, surely harbingers of arteriosclerotic heart disease. Heinrich Hermann Robert Koch died of a myocardial infarction on May 27, 1910, at Baden-Baden, a spa where he was recuperating from a respiratory infection. His cremated remains rest in the Robert Koch Institute.

Koch's Place in the History of Medicine

How can we chronicle Koch's accomplishments?

- He discovered or definitively characterized the pathogens we know as *Bacillus anthracis*, *Staphylococcus aureus*, *Mycobacterium tuberculosis*, and *Vibrio cholera*. Interestingly, in a field where most organisms are named for their discoverers, none of these bacteria bears his name. He, in fact, always referred to *M. tuberculosis* simply as the tubercle bacillus.
- He developed many important bacteriological techniques. Perhaps chief among them should stand plate cultures, which per-

mitted for the first time and still permit the isolation of organisms in pure culture from single colonies. He made similarly important contributions to microscopy and to sterilization procedures.

• In the end, he returned from microorganisms to the humans they attacked—not this time as the beloved physician of Rakwitz or Wollstein, but as the champion of public health.

Koch's death was noted by obituaries and tributes in medical and lay publications throughout the world. The British journal Lancet noted:

> Germany has to mourn the death of one of her greatest sons, Professor Robert Koch, who died in Baden-Baden on May 27th from arteriosclerosis and myocarditis. This is the heaviest loss which German science has sustained since the death of Virchow, and, as in the case of that great genius, the loss is not only that of Germany but of the whole world. For Koch was not only a savant of vast renown who has contributed more than any other man, perhaps including Virchow, to raise German science in esteem, but he was also a leader in the combat against the saddest diseases which threaten the welfare of the world. Not only his country but the whole world have received the benefits of his work, so that his death will be deplored everywhere throughout the civilised nations.[54]

The fiftieth and one hundredth anniversaries of Koch's description of the tubercle bacillus in 1882 sparked commemorative symposia and volumes in several scientific venues. I was privileged to edit the Koch Centennial Memorial volume published by the American Review of Respiratory Disease. At that time, I concluded my editorial about the discovery of the tubercle bacillus by stating, "We should recognize that this event had major importance not simply for phthisiology but for all of medicine."[55] I venture now that the passing of succeeding centuries will not diminish that estimation of the impact of Robert Koch on medicine and world health.

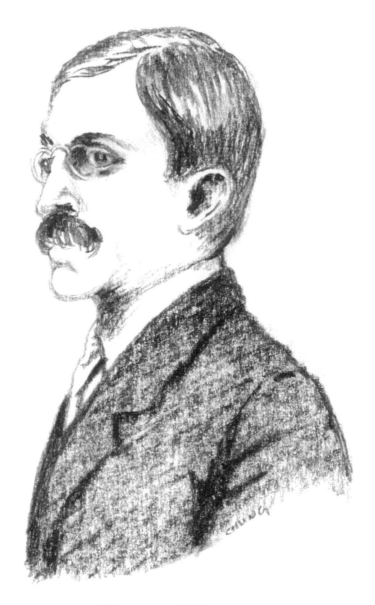

Hermann Michael Biggs

6

Hermann Michael Biggs
1859–1923
Pioneer of Public Health

The nineteenth century saw the dawning of new medical knowledge in many fields of medicine but none may have had as great an impact as the demonstration by Koch, Pasteur, and others that microorganisms are capable of causing disease. As we have seen in Chapter 1, the idea that tuberculosis and other diseases caused by these microorganisms could be transmitted from person to person was only reluctantly accepted by many physicians of the time, despite what now seems to be incontrovertible evidence supporting the concept. As early as the thirteenth century, physicians in Italy were writing of the infectious nature of tuberculosis, and by the late seventeenth century Italian cities had passed quarantine laws for this disease. Their ideas did not cross the Alps, however, and most northern Europeans and their American cousins considered tuberculosis to be a hereditary disease. Benjamin Marten's "animalcula" and Villemin's transmission of tuberculosis from one rabbit to another had little impact. Not until Koch's elegant demonstration of the tubercle bacillus was tuberculosis generally accepted as an infectious disease, and even then it took two or more decades to convince some outspoken skeptics.[1]

At about the same time, increasing awareness that many diseases could be spread from one person to another led to public demand for measures of protection and gave rise to the field of public health. The North American colonies enacted their first laws dealing with issues of public health in the mid seventeenth century, and the fledgling United States was less than a decade old when its congress enacted the first American quarantine laws.[2] As it became generally apparent that many infectious diseases were especially prevalent among immigrants and other disadvantaged persons and that epidemics might arise from these sources, the clamor for control of the perceived danger presented by these unfortunate and socially undesirable groups of people grew increasingly strident. The dawning of the nineteenth century saw the enactment of public health laws in several states. Within a few decades, a discipline of public health emerged in North America, and governments at various levels appointed health commissioners to implement and oversee public health measures to protect the citizenry by quarantine and other measures from the threat presented by sick individuals living within the community. In 1869 Massachusetts created the first state board of health, and New York followed in 1880. No health commissioner was more zealous or more forward-looking than Hermann M. Biggs of New York. Without question, he was the father of modern public health in North America.

Far above Cayuga's Waters

For thousands and thousands of years, glaciers scoured the face of much of North America. When they finally retreated from western New York State, they left behind the deep furrows that are today the scenically spectacular Finger Lakes, Lake Cayuga among them. Near the west shore of Lake Cayuga sits Trumansburg, a small town, originally Treman's Village, providing services to the rural area surrounding it. Hermann Michael Biggs was born in Trumansburg on September 29, 1859, the second of two children of Joseph Hunt Biggs and Melissa Pratt Biggs.[3] Both the Biggs and Pratt families were of English origin and had come to America as colonists in the seventeenth century. Hermann Biggs wrote to his older brother shortly after graduating from college about their ancestry, saying, "I do enjoy a good deal of solid satisfaction in knowing that if our ancestors were not all from the oldest and best families in the country, or from the nobility, they were at least honorable upright men, strong in themselves and in their convictions, which after all is the highest title to nobility."[4] The Biggs parents named their son to honor his uncle, Hermann Biggs, who served with distinction as a Brigadier General in the Civil War, and his grandfather Michael Biggs, who first brought the Biggs family to Trumansburg. Joseph Biggs was a successful merchant, with a store selling dry goods and hardware, and a pillar of his church and community, and the Biggs family lived comfortably in Trumansburg. If a town of only a thousand inhabitants could be said to have an aristocracy, then the Biggses certainly belonged to it.

Hermann Biggs's boyhood on the small farm that was the family homestead was a happy one. Winslow's biography contains a number of quotations from diaries kept by the boy, and they speak of rides on his pony, of hunting, and of sleighing and skating in the winter. A school paper written on the topic of snow gives insight into winter life in Trumansburg. "The boys think it is very useful for riding down hill and this winter they rode most of the time until the police stopped them. . . . It is also sometimes the cause of much trouble when it melts quickly causing the streams to rise carrying away bridges and dams on the streams as has been the case during the last month." In 1873, at the age of fourteen, Biggs wrote an essay entitled "Amusement." It reveals a serious side of the young man: "We are created with intellectual powers, with the ability to decide for ourselves, whether we will improve or neglect the talents given us by God. If we improve these talents to the best of our ability we are only performing part of the business of life, and that which our Creator requires for us. . . . If we neglect these talents, and spend our time in simply amusing ourselves we do not perform the duty for which we were created."[5] Hermann Biggs was growing up to be an upright citizen in small-town America. However, his talents would take him far beyond that small town.

Public schools in small American towns were limited at the time of Biggs's boyhood, and the Biggs parents did not think those in Trumansburg were adequate. Hermann attended the private Trumansburg Academy. Later he transferred to the Ithaca Academy. In 1877 Joseph Biggs died, and Hermann, then seventeen, dropped out of school and with John Daley, who had long worked as a clerk in the Biggs store, took over management of the family emporium. While successful in this endeavor, it did not satisfy him, and two years later he resumed his education. With his eye on Cornell University, which overlooked Lake Cayuga from its southeastern shore not far from Trumansburg, Biggs enrolled for one year at the Cornell University Preparatory School in Ithaca.

Hermann Biggs entered Cornell in 1879, only eleven years after that vibrant center of liberalism and learning enrolled its first students. Cornell

University was product of the dreams of Ezra Cornell and Andrew D. White, two close friends from Ithaca who were joined by their Unitarian religion and liberal social thought. Cornell had amassed a fortune building telegraph lines to transmit the signals emanating from Samuel Morse's new communications invention. He had little formal education. White was a Yale graduate imbued with liberal thought and the slavery abolitionist tradition. In 1862 White, who was to become the first president of Cornell University, had written a letter to the wealthy reformer and liberal abolitionist Gerritt Smith in which he envisioned a great university "where the most highly prized instruction may be afforded to all—regardless of sex or color." He went on to assert that this university should "afford an asylum for Science—where truth shall be sought for truth's sake, where it shall not be the main purpose of the Faculty to stretch or cut science exactly to fit `Revealed Religion.'" He hoped this university would become "a center from which ideas and men shall go forth to bless the nation during ages."[6] White's dream was realized when his friend Ezra Cornell offered to give "a farm of three hundred acres overlooking the village of Ithaca and Cayuga Lake . . . " and to "erect on the farm suitable buildings for the use of the college, and give an additional sum of money to make up an aggregate of three hundred thousand dollars. . . . "[7]

When Biggs entered the new university, not all of the buildings had been completed. A spirit of excitement permeated the new school. Biggs lived with an aunt in Ithaca, but he quickly became involved in campus life, joining a fraternity, playing the organ in the college chapel, and entering into the social life of the coeducational campus. His aunt was married to a doctor practicing in Ithaca, and this contact led the young student to become interested in studying medicine. Biggs carried far more courses than required, and by the end of his second year had finished most of his graduation requirements.

In the autumn of 1881, Biggs took leave and went to New York to enroll in the Bellevue Hospital Medical College. This medical school, which had been organized in 1861, had a commitment to community service dating from 1787, when the Almshouse Hospital, Bellevue Hospital's predecessor and the only public hospital in New York at the time, initiated a course of medical instruction that continued in one fashion or another from that time forward.[8] Although the Bellevue faculty was particularly distinguished for its expertise in surgery, these prominent men had interests that extended far beyond the operating theater. The three professors of surgery on the medical college faculty served on the Council on Hygiene and Public Health, which was organized in New York City in 1865. So also did Austin Flint, a distinguished clinician, and Edward Delafield, who was to achieve recognition as a pioneer pathologist. Thus, Hermann Biggs was almost certainly exposed to current thinking in public health during his early year at Bellevue. He returned to Cornell for the spring semester to finish his course work and receive his undergraduate degree in 1872.

A large panoply of experiences must have shaped Hermann Biggs's nascent career: boyhood in rural New York where mud in the spring was followed by dust in the summer and snow in the winter, where rugged individualism was a much admired trait, and where disease and lack of sanitation were the norms of life; two years of responsibility managing the family store; college at a new university steeped in liberal thought; enrollment in medical school in urban New York City crowded with tenements and sweat shops, disease ridden and lacking in simple measures of sanitation, and where garbage and offal were dumped on the streets and some eight thousand dead horses were left to decay in the streets each year;[9] and exposure to professors at the medical school who were concerned with issues of public health. Cornell required a thesis of its graduating students, and Biggs's paper was entitled "Sanitary Regulations and the Duty of the State in Regard to Public Hygiene." This paper reflects profound thought by the young man, and it is worth quoting at length from it, for it sets forth ideas that would remain at the head of Biggs's professional agenda throughout his life:

> The enjoyment of health, immunity from suffering and long life are the greatest temporal blessings that man can desire, and the questions of the attainment and maintenance of these are questions of no ordinary interest to the human race. Sanitary science is the science that pertains to health, and this affords a key to the correct answers to all these questions. There are certain natural and sanitary laws that regulate the functions of life, and a strict compliance with these would ensure to man a more uninterrupted enjoyment of health, exemption from many infirmities

and a prolonged existence. But we fall far short of the fulfillment of these requirements, and it is largely due to this that the allotted age of man is so much shortened.

It has been wisely said that "men are slow to learn the extent to which their destinies are in their own hands." They are astonished and incredulous when it is pointed out to them, that the most terrible maladies which have afflicted the human race are the direct and obvious consequences of the neglect or violation of the laws of health. But during the last few years the importance of hygienic laws has been more fully realized, especially by the medical profession, and by them has been brought prominently forward to the notice of the masses of the people.

Upon the recognition and careful observance of hygienic laws depend the healthy physical condition and so the prosperity not only of individuals and communities, but also of whole states and nations. More and more is this true as the density of population increases and great cities spring up, where vast numbers from the lowest grades of society are crowded together in small areas, which become the breeding places and hotbeds of disease.

But this age of neglect, carelessness and skepticism is rapidly passing away and all over the country can be seen the outcroppings of a genuine faith in the efficacy and importance of sanitary regulations, manifested by the establishment of health boards, and the critical investigation into the causes and sources of all endemic and epidemic diseases. We hail this as a great epoch in the history of preventive medicine pointing with no uncertain finger to a time not far distant, when all infections and contagious diseases shall be banished from our land, or so ameliorated in force and fatality, that they shall be despoiled of those characteristics which render them a terror in every household. . . .

A nation is made up of individuals, and so complex are these relations that each to some degree affects the whole. As the individuals are, so will the nation be. Not only is the physical condition of a people dependent on their sanitary surroundings, but their moral and intellectual condition is also largely determined by these same surroundings, for it has been truly said that "ignorance and vice are rather the effects than the causes of physical misery, and the surest mode of attacking them is to improve the physical condition of the lower classes, to abolish foul air, fouled water, foul lodgings and overcrowded dwellings, where morality is difficult and common decency impossible." When this is done not only will there be less of suffering and disease, but there will be also a higher standard of morality and intelligence throughout the country.

Health, loyalty, intelligence, morality and prosperity among a people demand as the essential conditions of their existence, pure air and pure water in abundance, sufficiently commodious dwellings and most of all cleanliness. To ensure the existence of these conditions everywhere among the people there should be some governmental inspection of the public health, there should be suitable national sanitary and quarantine regulations adopted and proper means for their enforcement provided. There should also be some way by which the people may be warned of the approach of those terrible contagious diseases such as cholera and yellow fever, and such foreign and internal quarantine measures adopted and enforced, so that we may never be compelled to look again with sorrow and regret upon the preventable desolation and death wrought by one of those great epidemics, that have devastated parts of our land so many times in the past.

"There was a time," says one of the best sanitarians in our State in a recent paper, "when fasting and prayer to avert disease on the one hand, and a faithless distrust of common sense on the other hand, were obstacles to the sanitary improvement of the masses and to the protection of the public health." When Lord Palmerston was waited on by a delegation of Scotch petitioners for the royal appointment of a day of fast, he surprised them by saying: "Go home and see that your towns and cities are freed from those causes and sources of contagion which, if allowed to remain, will breed pestilence and be fruitful in death, in spite of the prayers of a united but inactive people." This is the direction in which our present endeavors should be directed that the next steps in advance may be made possible. The people must be aroused to a fuller conviction of the importance of sanitary regulations. Lord Derby long ago declared that "no sanitary improvement worth the name will be effective whatever acts you pass or whatever powers you confer upon public officers unless you can create an intelligent interest in the matter among the people at large." But the people are becoming more and more alive to this subject of the public health and it may be truthfully said that in the last decade and a half greater advances have been made in public hygiene and more practical and valuable work done toward crushing out disease and remedying its causes than for many centuries before. Individuals, the states and the nation are becoming more and more aroused to the importance of prompt energetic and thorough action on this subject and we may legitimately look in the near future for still greater advances. Even now within the last month there has come to us across the waters from Germany the announcement of what promises to be the grandest discovery of the age—the discovery of a parasite as the cause of tuberculosis by Dr. Koch of Berlin. Professor Tyndall in an article upon this says "if the seriousness of a malady be measured by the number of victims then the most dreadful pests that have ravaged the world—plague and cholera included—must stand far behind the one now under consideration." Koch makes the startling statement that one-seventh of the deaths of the human race are due to the tubercular disease while fully one-third of those who die in active middle life are carried off by the same cause. Too much cannot be expected of the far-reaching consequences of this discovery, in it probably lies the solution of that problem so long regarded as unsolvable—the cure of tuberculosis. The *Medical News* says: "If Pasteur's culture experiments have led to the discovery of a method by which the poison of splenic fever is rendered harmless, and the disease prevented by the timely inoculation of the modified virus, may we not hope that the time is not distant when the ravages of consumption will be prevented by the inoculation of a modified bacillus?" No one can fail to be deeply impressed by the transcendent importance and far-reaching consequences of this discovery.

Then let us join in a cordial all hail to the coming centuries, to the time when zymotic diseases have become almost traditional, when life shall be prolonged and the enjoyment of health and immunity from suffering shall be almost universal through the advances in Preventive Medicine and the prevalence and observance of National Sanitary Regulations.[10]

This is a remarkable document to have come from the pen of a twenty-two-year-old college senior and first year medical student. Moreover, it presaged many of the guiding principles of Biggs's later career. "Public health can be purchased," he was wont to say. Moreover, he was guided by the tenet that the health of the poor was a necessary responsibility of the affluent. Finally, he never flinched in promulgating regulations imposing restrictions on individual behavior when doing so was in the interest of the health of the public at large.

Bellevue and Berlin

Hermann Biggs devoted the years 1882 to 1885 to his medical education. For his day his education was an excellent one, consisting largely of lectures and demonstrations by dedicated professors who were also leading practitioners in New York. Biggs was a diligent and superior student; he finished at the head of his class of 167. In March 1883 he sat for the examination for an internship at Bellevue Hospital, then the most prestigious clinical training available in New York. A letter from Austin Flint, Jr., advised him that he had been "successful in your examination for the position of interne in Bellevue Hospital and have passed with the rank of No. 1."[11]

Bellevue Hospital was a center of academic and clinical excellence, and clinician Edward G. Janeway and pathologist Francis Delafield dominated its clinical services and served as role models for the young Biggs.[12] Biggs was an outstanding student, impressing the faculty favorably. He became a protégé of Janeway, who later became the school's dean, and Janeway provided important support as Biggs's subsequent career developed.

The rapid advances in pathology and microbiology being made in Europe were well known in the halls of Bellevue. We have seen that Biggs cited Koch's discovery of the tubercle bacillus in his senior thesis at Cornell. This dramatic discovery, described in Chapter 5, and the international excitement surrounding it had a large impact on Biggs. During his internship year the young physician determined to go to Germany to further his studies, perhaps influenced by the visit to Bellevue of Dr. Paul Grawitz, one of the assistants of the eminent German pathologist, Rudolph Virchow. Armed with a dossier of introductory letters from Cornell and Bellevue, he presented himself first at the Berlin Physiological Institute and then at Greifswald. But Biggs was not happy in Germany. He was lonely and homesick, and he had less contact with the distinguished scientists of that land than he had hoped for. After six months he returned to New York.

New York City: The Battle against Infectious Diseases Is Joined

When Hermann Biggs sailed back through the Verrazano Narrows into New York Harbor he returned to a faculty appointment at Bellevue and its newly established Carnegie Laboratory. The Carnegie Laboratory, the first in North America to be dedicated to the study of disease by the methods of pathology and bacteriology, was originally designed for William Welch, who left New York to assume the leadership of the new Johns Hopkins School of Medicine in Baltimore before the laboratory was opened. Edward Janeway became the laboratory's director, and Biggs, who felt ill-prepared for the task, found himself in charge of the bacteriology laboratory. In his words, "When I came back from Germany in 1885 I was placed in charge of the work in the Carnegie Laboratory which had just been opened. There was practically no bacteriological work being done in this country, and while I knew very little about bacteriology, having found it almost impossible to get any instruction in the subject in Germany, yet I was obliged to commence giving instruction in it."[13]

Within one month of assuming his new post, Biggs found himself diverted to Plymouth, Pennsylvania, to investigate an epidemic of typhoid. Biggs and his coinvestigator A. A. Breneman quickly turned their attention to the town's water supply, which was drawn from four reservoirs, a stream, and a river, depending on the state of these various sources. They identified a house about sixty feet from one of the reservoirs where, "during the months of January, February, and March, one of the occupants was sick with a severe form of typhoid fever. During this time the excreta at night were thrown out back of the house, on the snow, and very near the stream. The weather was cold during these months, and this material was probably frozen fast where it was thrown, and rendered innoxious for the time. The latter part of March (from the 25th to the 30th) the weather was warm, and at this time these deposits, which had been accumulating through so long a period, were washed into the reservoir, containing then but a small quantity of water. At just this time (the evening of March 26th) the town began to draw its water supply from the reservoir again."[14] This travail should be viewed in the context of medical knowledge of that time. Typhoid had been known as an epidemic disease since ancient times, and William Budd had demonstrated that it could be transmitted by contaminated water in 1856, but its bacteriologic etiology was not established until 1884 by Georg Gaffky in Germany, only a year before Biggs's investigation in Plymouth.

While Hermann Biggs was establishing himself at Bellevue and, in the process, leading the medical revolution rooted in the sciences of bacteriology and pathology at that institution, another bright young physician was emerging into prominence at the College of Physicians and Surgeons, New York's other major medical school.[15] T. Mitchell Prudden, the son of a liberally minded Connecticut minister, studied chemistry and medicine at Yale University, receiving his medical degree in 1875.[16] He spent three months of his final year of medical school in New York City in the laboratory of Francis Delafield. After a year of internship in New Haven he went to Europe, as Biggs would do a decade later. He spent two years on that continent, sometimes in holiday traveling, other times in study at several German pathology laboratories. Upon his return, he accepted an appointment as Delafield's assistant in the pathology laboratory at the College of Physicians and Surgeons. During 1886 and 1887 Prudden and Biggs began a professional and personal relationship that lasted throughout their lives and that had an extraordinary impact upon public health in New York and throughout North America. In 1888 Biggs and Prudden along with Janeway and Horace P. Loomis were appointed consulting pathologists to the New York Department of Health.

Biggs's encounter with the Plymouth typhoid outbreak was scarcely over before he turned his attention to cholera. He wrote a scholarly review of the etiology of cholera and the identification by Koch of *Vibrio cholera*, then known as the comma bacillus, defending Koch's thesis at a time when it remained a source of substantial controversy.[17] Biggs's knowledge of this dread diarrheal disease was soon to be called upon, for the attention of New York's medical community and particularly of Drs. Joseph D. Bryant, who had been recently named Commissioner of Health, and William M. Smith, Health Officer of the Port, had become focused on the importation of cholera by passengers and crew members of ships arriving in New York.[18] On October 14, 1887, the steamship *Brittania* arrived from Marseilles with 408 steerage passengers. Three had died of intestinal illness during the voyage and others on the ship were ill at the time it docked. Biggs and Prudden obtained stool samples and cultured *V. cholera* from them, the first such isolation in North America. This event was only the beginning of Biggs's involvement with cholera. In August of 1892 an epidemic of cholera exploded in Hamburg, Germany, a major port of embarkation for immigrants destined for the United States, with nearly 18,000 cases reported during two months. New York responded by creating within its Health Department a Division of Pathology, Bacteriology, and Disinfection. Biggs was placed in charge of it as Chief Inspector; Prudden was named a consultant. Ships were quarantined and immigrants screened. Remarkably and almost certainly to Biggs's credit, no incidents of cholera transmission occurred in New York in the wake of this epidemic. There were two notable results of this episode. The world's first health department laboratory was established to provide diagnostic cultures, and this laboratory was of great importance for the city in establishing a safe water supply. Also, a principle of compromising individual liberties to protect the public health—in this case by quarantine and isolation of arriving passengers—was firmly established and converted into regulatory edict.

The limited outbreak of cholera on the *Brittania* was only a harbinger of events to come. On August 31, 1893, the *Moravia* docked in New York from Hamburg.[19] She was the first of seven ships, six from Hamburg, one from Liverpool, that Biggs dubbed "the cholera fleet." Twenty-two of the Moravia's passengers had succumbed to cholera at sea; an additional fifty-four persons met their demise from cholera during the voyages of the other ships that August and September. A number of secondary cases occurred, one as far away as Nevada, and Biggs and his colleagues imposed quarantines not only on the ships but on the houses of those who developed the disease in New York.

Biggs's stature in the New York medical community grew rapidly. New teaching assignments were given him, and he was soon recognized by both faculty and students as an outstanding professor. In April 1886, scarcely a year after his return from Germany, he received an appointment as visiting physician at Bellevue Hospital, and he found himself covering the service of his mentor Edward Janeway during the summer absence of that prominent physician. With this event, a busy clinical practice developed. Janeway considered Biggs an exceptional clinician and offered to bring him into his prosperous practice as his assistant, but Biggs turned down this offer in order to conserve his time for the laboratory. A trip to Paris to evaluate Pasteur's dramatic new and controversial treatment for rabies followed at the behest of Andrew Carnegie; the philanthropist, who had endowed Bellevue's laboratory, had read of Pasteur's success and wished to know more of it. The pace of Biggs's first years as a young physician and medical scientist in New York City was clearly extraordinary. It was not, as subsequent events were to demonstrate, exceptional for the energetic and talented Hermann Biggs.

Diphtheria was a major threat to the lives of New York's and the world's children. It had been identified as a distinct disease and given its name by the French physician Pierre Bretonneau early in the century, and in 1884 Friedrich Loeffler first described the corynebacterium that causes it. Émile Roux and Alexandre Yersin, working at Pasteur's institute in Paris, demonstrated that the disease was effected not by the bacillus itself but by a toxin that it produced, and in 1890 Emil von Behring, one of Koch's Berlin colleagues, first produced diphtheria antitoxin. The first Nobel Prize awarded in medicine or physiology went to him for this discovery, and within four years he was producing sufficient quantities of equine antiserum to treat large numbers of patients and convince the world that another dread infection had been conquered.[20] Hermann Biggs went to Europe in the summer of 1894. He visited von Behring at the Koch Institute, and he returned convinced that it was time to begin production of the miraculous antitoxin in New York, a project which he and Prudden soon brought to fruition. When the health department proved unwilling to commit funds for the purchases of horses in which to raise the antiserum, Biggs personally assumed financial responsibility for their acquisition.[21] Similarly, Prudden wished to raise diphtheria antiserum in horses at the College of Physicians and Surgeons. Told there was no money for horses, he purchased four. Told there was no place for them to be stabled, he paid for remodeling of a coal house into stables.[22] One of Prudden's horses was the first to develop high levels of antibody, and he shared the precious serum with Biggs and the Health Department.

Hermann Biggs did not stop with producing antitoxin for New York. He drafted legislation that was passed by the state legislature allowing the Health Department to sell this and other medical products. In Biggs's words, "The purpose of this bill was threefold: first, to make available diphtheria antitoxin for other cities which could not obtain it except at a very high price; second, to control and stabilize the price of these laboratory products; third to provide a fund which could be utilized by the Health Board for the establishment of a research laboratory in the Health Department."[23] Here we have another example of the farsighted and progressive wisdom of Hermann Biggs, a wisdom born of a vision that included the purchase of health for the public by the governmental agents of the public. Once again, the theme that public health can be purchased reemerged in Biggs's thinking, but this time he proposed a measure that would effectively limit private profiteering from this purchase.

Biggs was widely recognized both in his profession and as a public figure. His private practice grew steadily, and his cousin George Biggs joined him as his assistant. In 1892 he bought a house on West Fifty-eighth Street and began taking vacations in the Adirondacks. Later he purchased land in that wooded region and built there a retreat named Camp Trillium. About this time he made his own diagnosis of diabetes, and embarked on a program of strict dietary control but did not otherwise limit his activities. During the winter of 1896–97, Biggs courted Frances Richardson, to whom he had been introduced by one of his patients, and the following summer the couple announced their engagement. They were married on August 18, 1898, and honeymooned in Europe. Their marriage was an enduring, happy, and mutually supportive one.

In 1901, the notoriously corrupt politicians of Tammany Hall fell from power, and a new Republican administration took control of New York City. Biggs was offered a cabinet post as commissioner of health. Although he was urged by many to accept this position, he turned it down, agreeing instead to become chief medical officer to the Health Department, a post that he expected would leave him freer to pursue issues he felt to be important. Further recognition came to him that year when John D. Rockefeller asked him for advice on the formation of the Rockefeller Institute and named him to the original board of directors of that prestigious institution. In 1905 he was elected to the presidency of the National Tuberculosis Association (now the American Lung Association) and in the following year the presidency of the American Hygiene Association. Later in his life, in 1920, he would be elected president of the prestigious and elite American Association of Physicians, and in the same year he would receive an honorary degree from Harvard University.

Tuberculosis and Public Health

From his undergraduate days at Cornell when he had recognized the importance of Koch's identification of the microbe causing tuberculosis, Biggs had manifested an interest in that disease, and it would be in the establishment of programs to control tuberculosis that he would have his greatest impact on the emerging medical field of public health. In fact, tuberculosis was a public health problem of enormous importance in New York City, with greatest endemnicity in the crowded tenements housing large numbers of newly arrived immigrants. In 1891, the tuberculosis death rate in New York City was 307/100,000/year, a rate equalling or exceeding that of the most highly endemic countries today and approximately one-eighth the overall death rate of that year for the city. Pulmonary tuberculosis was the third most commonly reported cause of death in New York, trailing only behind diarrheal diseases and all diseases of the nervous system.[24] Hermann Biggs and his friends Mitchell Prudden and Henry Loomis felt that the time had come for an assault on this great white plague. They encouraged Health Commissioner Bryant to ask the Board of Health to commission a report on tuberculosis from the three of them. This report, submitted in 1889, only seven years after Koch's first isolation of the tubercle bacillus, focused on the infectious nature of the disease and was in its day truly pace-setting. It is worth reviewing this remarkable document in some detail. After an initial four paragraphs concerning the pathogenesis and bacteriologic etiology of tuberculosis, it continued:

> Tuberculosis is commonly produced in the lungs (which are the organs most frequently affected) by breathing air in which the living germs are suspended as dust. The material which is coughed up, sometimes in large quantities, by persons suffering from consumption contains these germs often in enormous numbers. This material when expectorated frequently lodges in places where it afterwards dries, as on the streets, floors, carpets, clothing, handkerchiefs, etc. After drying, in one way or another, it is very apt to become pulverized and float in the air as dust.
>
> It has been shown experimentally, that dust collected from the most varied points, in hospital wards, asylums, prisons, private houses, etc., where consumptive patients are present, or have been present, is capable of producing tuberculosis in animals when used for their inoculation. Such dust may retain for weeks its power of producing disease. On the other hand dust collected from rooms in institutions or houses that have not been occupied by tubercular patients does not produce the disease when used for the inoculation of animals.

These observations show that where there are cases of pulmonary tuberculosis, under ordinary conditions, the dust surrounding them often
contains the tubercle bacilli; and persons inhaling the air in which this
dust is suspended may be taking in the living germs. It should be distinctly understood that the breath of tuberculosis patients, and the moist
sputum, received in proper cups, are not elements of danger, but only
the dried and pulverized sputum. The breath and moist sputum are free
from danger, because the germs are not dislodged from moist surfaces
by currents of air. If all discharges were destroyed at the time of exit from
the body, the greatest danger of communication from man to man would
be removed.

It then follows, from what has been said, that tuberculosis is a distinctly preventable disease.

It is a well-known fact that some persons, and especially the members
of certain families, are particularly liable to tuberculosis, and this liability can be transmitted from parents to children. So marked and frequent
is this liability, and so frequent is the development of the disease in
particular families that the affection has long been considered hereditary. We now know that tuberculosis can only be caused by the entrance
of the germ into the body; and that this transmitted liability simply
renders the individual a more easy prey to the living germs when once
they have gained entrance.

The frequent occurrence of several cases of pulmonary tuberculosis in
a family is, then, to be explained, not on the supposition that the disease
itself has been inherited, but that it has been produced after birth by
transmission directly from some affected individual. Where the parents
are affected with tuberculosis the children from the earliest moments of
life are exposed to the disease under the most favorable conditions for its
transmission, for not only is the dust of the house likely to contain the
bacilli, but the relationship also between the parents and children, especially between mother and child, are of the close and intimate nature
especially favorable for the transmission by direct contact.

If, then, tuberculosis is not inherited, the question of prevention re-
solves itself, principally, into the avoidance of tubercular meat and milk,
and the destruction of discharges, especially the sputum, of tubercular
individuals. As to the first means of communication, those measures of
prevention alone answer the requirements which embrace the governmental inspection of dairy cows and of animals slaughtered for food,
and the rigid exclusion and destruction of all those found to be tubercular.

For the removal of the second means of communication, *i.e.*, the sputum of tubercular individuals—the problem is simple when the patients are confined to their rooms or houses; then wooden or pasteboard cups with covers should always be at hand for the reception of the sputum. These cups are supported in simple racks, and at least once daily, or more frequently if necessary, should be removed from the racks and thrown with their contents in the fire.

The disposition of the expectoration of persons who are not confined to their rooms or homes is a far more difficult problem. The expectoration certainly should not be discharged on the street, and the only practical means for its collection seems to be in handkerchiefs, which, when soiled, should at the earliest possible moment be soaked in a solution of 5 per cent of carbolic acid and then boiled and washed. Handkerchiefs thus soiled are exceedingly dangerous factors in distributing tubercle bacilli; for when the sputum becomes dry, it is easily separated in flakes from the cloth and then soon becomes pulverized and suspended as dust.

It becomes evident from what has been said, that the means which most certainly prevent the spread of this disease from one individual to another, are those of scrupulous cleanliness regarding the sputum. These means lie largely within the power of the affected individual. It is, furthermore, to be remembered that consumption is not always, as was formerly supposed, a fatal disease, but that it is in very many cases a distinctly curable affection.

An individual who is well on the road to recovery may, if he does not with the greatest care destroy his sputum, diminish greatly his chances of recovery by self-inoculation.

While the greatest danger of the spread of the disease from the sick to the well is in private houses and in hospitals, yet, if this danger is thoroughly appreciated it is for the most part quite under control, through the immediate destruction of the sputum and the enforcement of habits of cleanliness. But in places of public assembly, such as churches and theatres, particularly the latter, the conditions are different, and safety would seem to depend largely upon a dilution and partial removal of the floating and possibly dangerous dust by means of adequate ventilation.

Rooms in private houses and hospital wards that are occupied by phthisical patients should from time to time be thoroughly cleaned and disinfected, and this should always be done after they are vacated, before they are again occupied by other individuals.

Steamship companies should be obliged to furnish separate apartments for consumptive persons, so that no person in the exigencies of travel need be forced to share his room with one who might be a source of active danger to him.

We desire especially to emphasize the following facts:

1. That tuberculosis is a distinctly preventable disease.
2. That it is not directly inherited; and
3. That it is acquired by the direct transmission of the tubercle bacillus from the sick to the healthy, usually by means of the dried and pulverized sputum floating as dust in the air.

The measures, then, which are suggested for the prevention of the spread of tuberculosis are:

1. The security of the public against tubercular meat and milk, attained by a system of rigid official inspection of cattle;
2. The dissemination among the people of the knowledge that every tubercular person may be an actual source of danger to his associates, if the discharges from the lungs are not immediately destroyed or rendered harmless: and
3. The careful disinfection of rooms and hospital wards that are occupied or have been occupied by phthisical patients.

HERMANN M. BIGGS,
T. MITCHELL PRUDDEN,
HENRY P. LOOMIS,
Pathologists to the
New York City Health Department.
1889[25]

This document was remarkably prescient. It was also bold, perhaps brazen. It was written when many eminent physicians remained skeptical of Koch's work and held that tuberculosis was an inherited disease. Even among those who accepted the microbiologic etiology of tuberculosis, many believed that transmission was primarily by the oral route. As we have seen in Chapter 5, Koch and his disciple, Carl Flügge, had concluded that bacilli in aerosolized or dried respiratory secretions transmitted tuberculosis. Not until nearly two decades later, however, did Fidel perform experiments clearly demonstrating the aerial infectiousness of tubercle bacilli and Kolish show that organisms ingested or trapped in dust and placed in the upper airway were less infectious than airborne organisms.[26] The classical studies of William Firth Wells and Richard L. Riley, which firmly established the role of droplet nuclei in spreading tuberculosis from person to person were carried out in the 1930s and 1950s.[27]

Let us look at this report in light of our modern knowledge of tuberculosis. The first several paragraphs of the portion of the report quoted above deal with the pathogenesis and transmission of tuberculosis. Biggs and his colleagues clearly understood that tuberculosis is an airborne infection. They correctly noted that familial occurrences were due not to inherited disease but to inherited susceptibility to disease following infection; it "renders the individual a more easy prey to the living germs when once they have gained entrance." Max Lurie, whose work firmly established this concept experimentally, was only six years old at the time and would not begin his elegant studies in rabbits for another quarter century.[28] Later in the report the authors correctly note the importance of transmission in the relatively confined environment of the home. However, the emphasis of the report on dust particles as fomites is misplaced, although the report does state that "germs are not dislodged from moist surfaces by currents of air." Incorrectly and in the context of considering dust and other fomites, the report says that "the breath . . . [is] free from danger."

Biggs and his two colleagues then turned their attention to public health measures for the prevention of the spread of tuberculous infection. They correctly noted that "discharges" are most easily contained and destroyed "at the time of exit from the body," a concept that led to enjoining millions of tuberculous patients and the public to "cover your cough." They called for the inspection of dairy and beef cattle, a measure that had already been championed by the medical community. They perceptively noted that the danger of transmission in public places could be reduced by adequate ventilation. On the other hand, they called for methods of decontamination that were unnecessarily harsh. One can wonder how many times one would be able to adorn a vest pocket or sleeve with a handkerchief that "at the earliest possible moment [after each use was to] be soaked in a solution of 5 per cent of carbolic acid and then boiled and washed." Finally, the danger of aerial self-inoculation described in the report simply does not exist.

The report of Biggs, Prudden, and Loomis was not uniformly welcomed by the contemporary medical community, many of its members being unconvinced of the infectious nature of tuberculosis. And the report did lead to sanitary measures that, by any modern standard, were extreme.[29] However, within two months the Board of Health had published a circular which marked the initiation of the first public education campaign for the conquest of any disease. It read:

Rules to be Observed for the Prevention of the Spread of Consumption

By observing the following rules the danger of catching the disease will be reduced to a minimum:

I.—Do not permit persons having consumption to spit on the floor or on cloths, unless the latter be immediately burned. The expectoration of persons suspected to have consumption should be caught in earthen or glass dishes containing the following solution: Corrosive sublimate,[30] seven grains; water, one pint, and finally thrown into the sewer or burned.

II.—Do not sleep in a room occupied by a person who has consumption. The living room of a consumptive patient should have as little furniture as practicable. Hangings should be carefully avoided. The use of carpets and rugs ought always to be avoided.

III.—Do not fail to wash thoroughly the eating utensils of a person who has consumption as soon after eating as possible, using boiling water for the purpose.

IV.—Do not mingle the unwashed clothing of a consumptive person with similar clothing of other persons. The soiled clothing of a consumptive person should be removed at once, put in boiling water for forty-five minutes, or otherwise disinfected.

V.—Do not fail to catch the bowel discharges of a consumptive person with diarrhea in a vessel containing corrosive sublimate seven grains to water one pint.

VI.—Do not fail to consult the family physician regarding the social relations of persons suffering from suspected consumption.

VII.—Do not permit mothers suspected of having consumption to nurse their offspring.

VIII.—Household pets (animals or birds) are quite susceptible to tuberculosis, therefore, do not expose them to persons afflicted with consumption; also, do not keep but destroy at once all household pets suspected of having consumption, otherwise they may give it to human beings.

IX.—Do not fail to cleanse thoroughly the floors, walls and ceilings of the living and sleeping rooms of persons suffering from consumption at least once in two weeks.

> By order of the Board.
> CHARLES G. WILSON, *President*
> EMMONS CLARK, *Secretary.*[31]

As with the earlier report, the emphasis of this document on infectious fomites was misplaced by today's standards, leading to unnecessary and almost punitive measures. Pets are known today generally not to be susceptible to tuberculosis. Yet, it was not until 1964 that John Chapman and Margaret Dyerly clearly showed that the residences of tuberculous patients in Dallas, Texas did not remain infectious after their removal from the home (Chapter 1).[32] However, the focus on preventing transmission of infection was appropriately placed. Public enthusiasm for it was high in New York (although not necessarily elsewhere), and more than 2,500 persons were arrested in that city for spitting in public places.[33]

Not all of Biggs's ideas for the control of tuberculosis were easily accepted, but he persisted in his advocacy. In 1893, Biggs, Prudden, and Loomis urged the New York City Board of Health to commission a report on tuberculosis, and on November 28 the board formally requested such a report of Dr. Hermann M. Biggs, Chief Inspector of the Division of Pathology, Bacteriology and Disinfection. Biggs was ready, and his report was delivered on the same day. It concluded with the following recommendations:

> I would, therefore, recommend, first, that there be systematically disseminated among the people by means of circulars, publications, etc., the knowledge that every tubercular person may be a source of actual danger to his associates, and his own chances of recovery diminished, if the discharges from the lungs are not immediately destroyed or rendered harmless.
>
> Second, that all public institutions, such as asylums, homes, hospitals, dispensaries, etc., be required to transmit to the Board of Health the names and addresses of all persons suffering from pulmonary tuberculosis within seven days of the time when such persons first come under observation.

Third, that special Inspectors be assigned to duty for the investigation of this disease, and whenever the Department has become aware of the existence of families or premises where tuberculosis exists, or has recently existed (as in case of death or removal), it shall be the duty of these Inspectors to visit such premises and deliver proper circulars, and give suitable information, to the persons residing there, and take such specific measures of disinfection as are required in each case.

Fourth, that the Board urge upon hospital authorities the importance of separation, so far as possible, in the hospitals of this city, of persons suffering from pulmonary tuberculosis from those affected with other diseases, and urge that proper wards be set apart for the treatment of this disease.

Fifth, that the Department of Charities and Correction of this city be requested to provide a hospital to be known as "The Consumptive Hospital," to be used for the exclusive treatment of this disease, and that, so far as practicable, all inmates of the various institutions under its care suffering from tuberculosis be transferred to this hospital.

Sixth, that the Health Department undertake the bacteriological examination of the sputum for diagnosis in every case of pulmonary disease of doubtful character in hospitals or private dwellings or tenement-houses, where the physician in attendance desires that this should be done. This procedure to be carried out with a view to obtain [sic] definite knowledge upon which the proper sanitary surveillance of those suffering from tuberculosis can be based.

Seventh, that all physicians practicing their professions in this city be requested to notify this Board of all cases of pulmonary tuberculosis coming under their professional care.[34]

Biggs's recommendations that institutions be required and physicians requested to report cases of tuberculosis was pioneering and a revolutionary idea for its time. It created a fire-storm of angry criticism in the medical community. Most physicians, many of whom still did not believe tuberculosis to be contagious, considered it an intrusion upon their rights as practitioners. An editorial in the *Medical Record*, a leading medical journal of New York City at that time, railed against Biggs:

THE HEALTH BOARD AND
COMPULSORY REPORTS
The profession of this city will be surprised to learn that the Health Board has finally declared that all cases of pulmonary tuberculosis, pub-

lic or private, shall be reported to its sanitary bureau, on the plausible ground that the disease in question is pronouncedly dangerous to public health. With every desire to interpret the motives of the Board in the most liberal spirit, the conviction forces itself upon us that the compulsory step taken is a mistaken, untimely, irrational, and unwise one. The medical profession is not yet prepared to endorse the radical measures proposed. While admitting that pulmonary tuberculosis in a very limited degree may be contagious, that the public should be properly educated in regard to the demonstrated causes of infection, that the spitting nuisance should be abolished, and every reasonable means should be used to the end of preventing the spread of the disease, it appears evident that the advisers of the Board have assumed, in the present instance, a position so far in advance of the general opinion of the profession as to the real necessity of the measure that a serious question of authority may be brought to the surface of general discussion. This latter will be a matter to be deplored, inasmuch as the profession has generally, in questions of ordinary policy, seconded any laudable endeavors of the Board to stamp out dangerously infectious diseases. The real strength of the Board depends upon such backing, but when the line is drawn too tightly, when too much authority is assumed, and too many orders are give, a reaction is likely to occur. The argument upon which the action is based is very much one-sided, and calculated, in the interest of a few of the workers in the board, to alarm the public unduly, to place a large number of patients under public jurisdiction, and to inflict unnecessarily extra burdens upon the medical attendant.

The real obnoxiousness of this amendment to the sanitary code is its offensively dictatorial and defiantly compulsory character. It places the Board in the rather equivocal position of dictating to the profession and of creating a suspicion of an extra bid for public applause by unduly magnifying the importance of its bacteriological department.[35]

The College of Physicians of Philadelphia, faced with the prospect of a similar proposal in their city in 1894, articulated a widely held medical opinion, "that the attempt to register consumptives and to treat them as the subjects of contagious disease would be adding hardship to the lives of those unfortunates, stamping them as the outcasts of society."[36] On the other hand, the lay press and many medical leaders supported Biggs. On February 13, 1894, the Board of Health accepted Biggs's report and tuberculosis notification became a fact. Between March

1 and December 31 of that year, 4,166 cases of tuberculosis were reported.[37] In 1897 the notification requirements were strengthened when the city adopted an ordinance declaring that, "tuberculosis is . . . an infectious and communicable disease, dangerous to the public health. It shall be the duty of every physician in this city to report to the Sanitary Bureau in writing . . . every person having such disease who has been attended by or has come under the observation of such physician for the first time within one week of such time."[38]

Biggs fully understood the radical nature of his aggressive approach to tuberculosis control. He knew that he faced opposition from many sources, but he was convinced his ideas were correct and that they would engender public support. In an address to a meeting of the British Medical Association in Montréal he said, "We are prepared, when necessary, to introduce and enforce, and the people are ready to accept, measures which might seem radical and arbitrary, if they were not plainly designed for the public good, and evidently beneficial in their effects. Even among the most ignorant of our foreign-born population, few or no indications of resentment are exhibited to the exercise of arbitrary powers in sanitary matters."[39] In one of his last acts as New York City General Medical Officer, Biggs submitted to the Commissioner of health a paper in which he stated:

> Of the various features of the antituberculosis work, none is more fundamentally important than notification and registration of cases; and none has been more misunderstood or opposed by the medical profession. In spite of almost innumerable objections at first urged, it has finally been realized that no adequate control of tuberculosis can be effected without such notification, and the objectors one by one have been silenced. To a large extent, objections of this sort come from those who fear innovations of any kind, and who refuse absolutely to adopt new procedures. In a vague way they feel that notification will have some dire consequences and they conjure up all sorts of imaginary evils, of a kind that never materialize.[40]

Tuberculosis case reporting soon followed elsewhere in North America and its importance was widely recognized. A letter from Robert Koch, by then a professor of hygiene in Berlin, written on May 26, 1901, read:

Honored Colleague:

You have been good enough to send me, through the courtesy of the American Consulate in Berlin, the existing regulations and other literature in regard to measures taken for the control of tuberculosis and other communicable disease in New York—for which I desire to express my most cordial thanks. We have much to learn from what in my opinion appear to be procedures adapted in an extraordinarily practical and adequate manner to the control of tuberculosis as you have carried them out in New York, since I believe that for us, too, the time has come to do something more in the control of this disease than has hitherto been possible. Public opinion is now ripe for such action so that the opportunity has come to secure the fundamental regulation for compulsory notification. In connection with the preparation of a law dealing with the control of communicable diseases in general, which is now in course I hope to secure the inclusion in this country of the compulsory reporting of such cases of pulmonary tuberculosis as are in a communicable state although I am finding strong opposition to such a step. To meet this opposition I wish to cite the example of the free American people who have of their own free will accepted the limitation of their own liberties in the interest of the public health. I wish it were also possible to demonstrate to these people unquestionable results of such a policy, that is to say a definite decrease of tuberculosis in the state of New York. But it is as yet too early for that. If, however, you should have any evidence of this sort I beg you to send it to me as it would prove of the greatest value.

> With highest respect,
> Yours,
> R. KOCH.[41]

At an international congress on tuberculosis in London in 1901, which Biggs was unable to attend, his mentor and friend Edward Janeway read a paper written by Biggs and describing the New York tuberculosis reporting experience. Following the presentation, William Osler, probably the most widely respected clinician of the time, moved a vote of thanks to Biggs, stating, in part:

I would ask any of you who are interested in this question of compulsory registration to read the reports of the city of New York for the past six or eight years. They form an object lesson on this work, which is of the greatest practical value to the communities, not only in the United

States, but to cities throughout the world. It gives me the greatest plea-
sure to move this vote of thanks to Dr. Biggs.[42]

In 1905, Biggs's medical colleagues accorded him further recognition by
electing him to the presidency of the National Association for the Study
and Prevention of Tuberculosis, today the American Lung Association.

With public education and case reporting in place as measures for
the control of tuberculosis in New York City, Biggs turned his attention
to the provision of hospital care for afflicted persons, the fifth of his
November 28, 1893, recommendations to the New York City Board of
Health. Sanatorium care had become accepted as therapeutically beneficial to persons with tuberculosis, and these institutions were rapidly
being founded in many locations.[43] The Health Department had already opened the first city run dispensary for indigent tuberculosis patients and opened the Riverside Hospital on North Brother Island in
the East River, but more was needed in a more suitable location. For
years Biggs lobbied the state legislature for funds, and finally in 1905
money was appropriated for the purchase of 1,200 acres of land, and
the world's first municipal sanatorium was opened in Otisville, New
York, sixty miles northwest of Manhattan in the Shawnagunk Mountains, for the treatment of tuberculosis patients from New York City.
Once again, Hermann Biggs had marched in the van of progressive
thought in the use of public funds to secure the public health.

Much as Biggs deserves credit for the founding of the first public municipal tuberculosis sanatorium, it should not be forgotten that earlier
special facilities for the inpatient care of consumptives were established
in Mammoth Cave, Kentucky, in 1842; in Boston, Massachusetts, in 1857;
and in Germany in 1859. Edward Livingston Trudeau opened his
Adirondack Cottage Sanitorium in Saranac Lake, New York, in 1884.[44]
There were, moreover, considerable segments of the medical and political
communities who viewed tuberculosis as a disease of undesirable persons
whose banishment would profit society in many ways, and these persons
were eager to embrace Biggs's proposal with less than altruistic motives.[45]

New York State Health Commissioner

The election of William Sulzer as governor of New York State in 1912
ushered in a tumultuous period in the politics of the state and also

dramatic changes in American public health and the life of Hermann Biggs. Sulzer served less than one year before a scandal broke over his campaign finances. He was impeached and removed from office. However, during his brief tenure he secured for the state a forward-looking law creating a Public Health Council and Commissioner of Public Health to be appointed by the governor and empowered to enact a sanitary code for the state, excluding New York City. This radical step removed the health department from the machinations of the state legislature, but it did not depoliticize it. Sulzer asked Biggs to accept the position of Health Commissioner. Biggs, whose health was declining, refused the nomination. Sulzer nominated him again, and again Biggs demurred. Martin H. Glynn, who moved up from lieutenant governor to governor following Sulzer's departure, again asked Biggs to serve and announced that if Biggs did not accept he would appoint a prominent opponent of many of the forward-looking measures Biggs had fought for. With that, Biggs capitulated, and in 1914 he became State Commissioner of Health, resigning his position in New York City, and he recruited a dynamic cadre of colleagues to join him working for New York State.[46]

It did not take long for Biggs to make his mark. A smallpox epidemic raged in Niagara Falls. New York State had enacted a quarantine law for smallpox in 1778 and a law providing for compulsory vaccination of school children in 1860, but these laws had been strongly resisted by civic and medical leaders in Niagara Falls and the surrounding areas of western New York State. An average of 613 cases of smallpox had occurred during each of the seven preceding years. Niagara Falls was identified in newspaper accounts nationally as a "plague spot." Despite this, no vaccinations were carried out by local health officials, and the mayor responded to these reports that the "statement that smallpox is epidemic in Niagara Falls [is] absolutely without foundation. Not a single case of the disease in the city." In fact, at the time the mayor spoke, the local health officer knew of ten cases. Additional cases occurred, and by January 1914 there were 75 known cases, and desultory vaccination efforts were beginning.[47]

The day after taking office, Biggs sent a health officer to investigate, and within a week Biggs had told him that "more radical measures must be taken in Niagara Falls to suppress the epidemic of smallpox. The

people of other portions of the state must be protected against the fol-
lies of any local community at whatever cost may be necessary." Biggs
outlined a series of tough quarantine measures and closures of public
places and asked his representative to "request the mayor to call a meeting of the local authorities, prominent business men and manufactur-
ers" to advise them of his readiness to "absolutely isolate Niagara Falls
from its relations with other portions of the country" if necessary. Biggs
secured the agreement of the New York Central Railroad to stop providing rail service to Niagara Falls, and posters were printed to advise
the public of the absence of rail service. A committee of business leaders
of Niagara Falls telephoned Biggs to protest the economic impact of the
proposed measures and to ask him for time to allow them to confer
with their colleagues. "I will give you one hour and no more," Biggs
replied. Within the hour the city capitulated and prepared for a mass
vaccination program and appropriate quarantine of cases. The epidemic
was aborted over the next two months, but not until 550 people had
contracted smallpox, with spread to 21 other communities in the state.

With Hermann Biggs at the helm, the New York State Health Department would never be the same. It adopted a motto, "Public health
is purchasable. Within natural limitations any community can determine its own death rate," reflecting a theme that ran through the mind
of Hermann Biggs throughout his life of public service. In the letter of
transmittal accompanying his first annual report to the governor, Biggs
wrote, "These discoveries [of scientific medicine] promise many benefits which are as yet very incompletely realized, and open new fields of
activity as yet almost untouched. It is the earnest desire of my associates
and myself, through the State Department of Health, to render them
available in a greater degree than in the past, for the prevention of disease and the prolongation of life."[48]

The health department set itself the task of saving 25,000 lives within
five years; Biggs was by nature a goal setter. Infant health was promoted,
and public health nursing brought to prominence. A poliomyelitis epidemic in 1916 and the great influenza epidemic of 1917 and 1918
provided challenges that were beyond the reach of medical science of
the day, and Biggs's role was largely limited to preaching calm and common sense. Not surprisingly, tuberculosis was high on Biggs's agenda,
and clinics and tuberculosis hospitals were built in many counties. Al-

though Hermann Biggs was known to his colleagues as "a diplomat, preferring to accomplish results by persuasion, education and example rather than by aggressive methods,"[49] However, he had to work in the arena of New York State politics, often marked by corruption, and Biggs's tenure was not always easy. Efforts by Republican politicians—Biggs was a Democrat—to remove him from office were mounted on several occasions, but Biggs had strong support within the medical community and the public, and he survived these attacks. Charles-Edward A. Winslow, one of his close associates, said of Biggs and his tenure as state health commissioner in a tribute written after his death, "He was a great executive, knowing how to select his subordinates, how to inspire them, how to let them alone, and how to check them up with an almost uncanny instinct when anything was going wrong. . . . He was a great man—comprehending, wise, courageous, loyal, master of himself and of the situations which confronted him."[50] The New York sanitary code of 1913, which created the Public Health Council and empowered the post of Health Commissioner, gave to the council the authority to establish sanitary regulations with the effect of law, and Biggs and his colleagues on the council were not reluctant to use this power. Twenty-four diseases were designated communicable, and in March 1916 reporting of these diseases by physicians, dispensaries, hospitals and other institutions became mandatory in New York State. The regulations provided for isolation and quarantine of infectious patients with these diseases.[51]

When the drum roll of World War I swept across France in 1914, tuberculosis exploded in its wake. In 1917 Biggs was sent by the Rockefeller Foundation to survey the situation. His report led to support by the foundation of a major antituberculosis program in that country. At home, Biggs was concerned that a major epidemic of sexually transmitted diseases might erupt with the return of troops from Europe;[52] in fact, this did not occur. In the postwar years Biggs joined a conference at Cannes of the League of Red Cross Societies, which dated its origins to 1863 and which later became the International Red Cross. In the summer of 1920 he served briefly as the Red Cross's General Medical Director in Geneva.

The crusade against tuberculosis waged by Hermann Biggs and his associates in New York was viewed by Biggs as his greatest accomplishment. "The activities of the Tuberculosis Division [of the State Department of

Health] . . . ," he wrote, "comprised essentially the determination of the needs and facilities for effective campaigning against tuberculosis, the initiation and demonstration of preventive measures and the stimulation of their adoption by the local communities of the State. . . . During the year [1919] 25,136 cases of tuberculosis were reported to the Division. . . . The pronounced improvement in the sanitary supervision of cases noted during 1918 was more striking during 1919. . . . "[53] At that time, Biggs noted, there were 37 public hospitals in the state exclusive of those of New York City and seven additional private tuberculosis hospitals. Tuberculosis dispensaries were opened throughout the state, and continuing medical education courses instituted in many localities for health professionals caring for tuberculous patients. Promotional literature on tuberculosis was prepared and published. In 1920 a mobile chest radiology unit was purchased and put into service.

Hermann Biggs was forward looking and concerned for the health of all of the citizens of New York. He noted that many areas of the state did not have adequate numbers of physicians or medical facilities:

> The situation with regard to medical service in rural communities is steadily growing more serious. The first intimation of the existing conditions came to the Department through the discovery that a very large number of local health officers were the only physicians in their respective municipalities and that the rural health officers as a class were men well advanced in years. The additional attention directed to the situation by the epidemics of poliomyelitis and influenza and by the war, and the continually increasing number of requests for assistance in securing physicians for municipalities which were without medical service led to a careful investigation by the Department. This revealed a problem of such character and extent as to require that steps be taken at once for its solution if the fundamental and vital health interests of the State are to be effectively guarded.
>
> The number of physicians in practice in small towns and rural districts is steadily decreasing while the population continues slowly to increase. At the same time the physicians in the rural sections of the State as a whole have been in practice on an average for over twenty-five years, and the number of recent graduates taking up rural practice is far less each year than the number of rural practitioners who die or retire or move into the cities. There were a large number of municipalities (over

325) without a single physician, who has been in practice less than 25 years. When residents of rural districts become seriously sick, owing to the lack of physicians, nurses and domestic servants, it is becoming more and more imperative that if they are to receive even ordinary care they shall be removed to a hospital. About one-fourth of the up-state counties have no hospitals within their limits and where hospitals are available they are often inadequate, and generally have not the facilities to give the best kind of medical and surgical service. The American College of Surgeons has approved but fourteen of the thirty-four larger hospitals located in the State outside of New York city.[54]

Problems such as this have received much attention in recent years, and legislative efforts have been made a national, state, and local levels to remediate them. But in the early 1920s a laissez-faire approach to the health needs of the medically underserved was the norm. Not for Biggs, however. He proposed a radical health bill for New York. In the words of his colleague, friend, and biographer Charles-Edward A. Winslow, "The purpose of the proposed bill was not only to develop school medical service, public health nursing and public health education throughout the state and to coordinate all existing public health activities within specified rural or semi-rural areas; but also `to encourage and provide facilities for an annual medical examination to detect physical defects and disease;' to assist the local practitioner of medicine by bacteriological and chemical laboratory diagnoses, x-ray facilities and expert clinical consultation service; and `to provide for the residents of rural districts, for industrial workers and all others in need of such service, scientific medical and surgical treatment, hospital and dispensary facilities, and nursing care, at a cost within their means or, *if necessary, free* [italics added].'"[55] That this forward-looking idea was resisted by organized medicine is no surprise; it would be nearly three-quarters of century before Medicaid, Medicare, and health-maintenance organizations would come to prominence in the American health care arena. Enabling legislation was introduced and defeated in the state legislature. It was reintroduced the following year, supported by Biggs in an emotional address to the legislature, and again defeated. But Biggs continued his campaign, and bit by bit small pieces of legislation were enacted. In 1923 New York enacted laws permitting state funding in support of county public health programs, including clinics and hospitals.

Biggs's health was failing. A cholecystectomy at the Mayo Clinic in 1920 produced some improvement, but he was increasingly frail. The letter of transmittal accompanying his last annual report of the State Department of Health, which was submitted five months before he died, was a scant two sentences long.[56] Previous transmittal letters had been masterful summaries of current conditions and proposals for their amelioration.

He made his last public address to a National Conference on Social Work on May 23, 1923, and at that time he reviewed his accomplishments in New York State and closed with a remarkable manifesto:

> Some of the most important health objectives of the next twenty years then may be briefly summarized as follows:
>   1. Establishing the custom of obtaining periodic physical examinations of every individual made by competent physicians.
>   2. Provision of systematic instruction in elementary physiology and hygiene and in health habits in the primary and secondary schools, and more extensive instruction in the normal schools and universities.
>   3. Further reduction in the death rate from the common infective diseases, such as tuberculosis, diphtheria, typhoid fever, scarlet fever, diarrheal diseases of infancy, etc.
>   4. Postponement of the age at which death occurs from the cardiovascular diseases and the other diseases of later life, through physical examination and instructions as to methods for retarding or arresting their progress.
>   5. Continued efforts, through research, to solve the problems connected with the causation and prevention of the acute respiratory diseases and cancer.
>   6. Continued efforts to prevent and cure certain diseases of nutrition and metabolism, such as diabetes, scurvy, rachitis and gout.
>   7. The prevention by education and law enforcement of new infections in the venereal diseases, and provision for more adequate treatment of syphilis.
>   8. The extension of the educational work of the public health authorities as a most effective means to promote the preservation of health and the prevention of disease.
>   9. Better and more extensive organization of the prenatal, maternity and infant work, and the care of the preschool child.

10. The extension of the work in mental hygiene and oral hygiene, including the ample facilities for treatment.
11. The efficient development and extension of medical school inspection, and its follow-up with the provision of adequate facilities for the treatment of the diseases and defects found in school children."[57]

Biggs closed this presentation with two remarkable sentences that are not part of his declaration of goals. They caution that care would be needed in assessing the outcomes of the measures he proposed. They are harbingers of the more sophisticated approaches to public health that were soon to be championed by a new cadre of epidemiologists under the leadership of Wade Hampton Frost (Chapter 8). Biggs said, "We must look to a decrease in the specific death rates in the future and not expect continuous and material reductions in the crude death rates. On the contrary, if the population begins to reach a stable equilibrium, and birth rates continue to fall and approach the death rates, the crude death rates will tend to increase as has been the case in France."[58]

Public health professionals would address Biggs's objectives in the following years, and we can now look back on their achievement with pride and satisfaction. Hermann Biggs pointed the way. He died of pneumonia on June 28, 1923, leaving behind a changed world and a vision for further change.

What was the enduring legacy of Hermann Michael Biggs? A vision of a healthier world purchased by activist agencies of the public. What were his contributions to the crusade against tuberculosis? Diagnostic services for all. Treatment for all. Case reporting. These innovations of Hermann Biggs remain to this day the foundation of tuberculosis control. In a tribute to his friend and colleague, Simon Flexner, Director of the Rockefeller Institute, wrote:

Doctor Hermann M. Biggs is dead. . . .

To those devoted to the improvement of the public health, Dr. Biggs stood for more than a quarter of a century as the highest, the most effective, and most resourceful exponent of the effort.

But although Dr. Biggs is dead, his work lives. . . . Never indeed has that work, and the spirit behind it, been so strong. . . . [59]

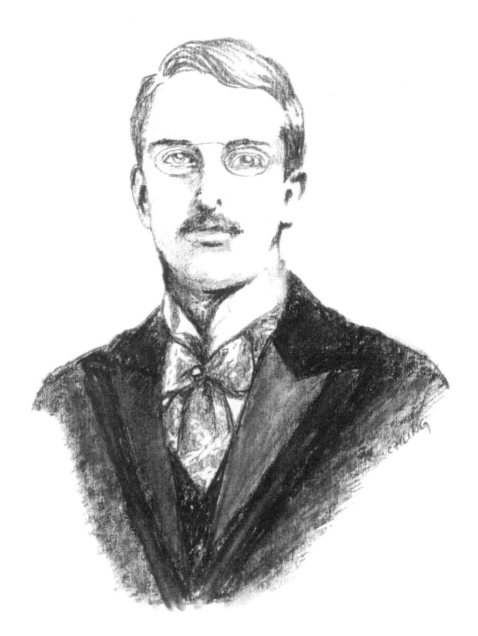

Clemens Freiherr von Pirquet

7

Clemens Freiherr von Pirquet
1874–1929
Pioneer of Immunology

As the later centuries of the second millennium unfolded, medical knowledge became centered in a number of European cities with major university faculties. These centers shifted. Vesalius's Padua yielded to Paris, home of Corvisart, Laennec, and Pasteur. Paris then gave way to Berlin, home of Henle, Virchow, Koch, von Behring, and Ehrlich. Toward the end of the nineteenth century, medical scholars began to concentrate in Vienna. Vienna, the city of Mozart and Strauss, the city of the River Danube, was founded in antiquity by Celts and became the easternmost outpost of Christian Europe confronting Muslim Turks. As the twentieth century dawned, Vienna was a center of both commerce and the arts. With more than one and one-half million inhabitants, it was the fourth-largest city of Europe. It and its citizens were known for conviviality as well as cultural sophistication. Vienna's university, founded in 1365, was a center of learning famous throughout the world. There, clinical medical specialties arose, and physicians from across the world came to study and improve both their clinical skills and the arrays of diplomas on the walls of their offices. It was in this hub of medical thought that Clemens von Pirquet would make his pioneering contributions to medicine.

The work of Pasteur and Koch had created the field of microbiology. Virchow and other pathologists had learned to exploit histologic examinations to reveal details of disease processes. John Snow had brought epidemiological thinking to medicine. Emil von Behring had introduced life-saving antiserum therapy for diphtheria. The stage was set for new dramas in the arena of infectious diseases and immunologic responses to them. Clemens von Pirquet stepped to the center of this proscenium. Sometimes considered the father of allergy, he would be better denominated the father of immunology, for he was the pioneer who was responsible for much of the thought that underlies this modern science. He became the leading pediatrician of Vienna, perhaps of the world, but his greatest and most enduring contributions were to the understanding of immune processes. Clearly a man of genius, his candle burned brightly during his youth and was tragically prematurely extinguished. Keats wrote almost all of his remarkable poetry during a single year. Gioacchino Rossini, whose life spanned three-quarters of a century, wrote all of his thirty-eight operas in nineteen years, none being composed during the ensuing forty years. The pioneering abstract painter Jackson Pollock produced his greatest paintings in a three-year creative burst that was followed by five years of almost no output, which ended in his early death. Similarly, Clemens von Pirquet was most productive during a short period of about five youthful years.

Freiherr

The map of Europe prior to the French Revolution and the Napoleonic wars was very different from that familiar today. The Austrian Empire included not only modern day Austria and large portions of eastern Europe, but also much of modern Belgium, including Liege, a city on the Meuse River near the eastern border of the country. The Pirquet family lived in Liege and was prosperous, but the capture of the city in 1794 by the French revolutionary army left the family penniless. Pierre Martin Pirquet, Clemens's grandfather, joined a military regiment loyal to the Austrian Empire. When this regiment joined the Prussian and British armies facing Napoleon's grande armée at Waterloo in 1815, Pierre Pirquet distinguished himself by his bravery. He was decorated and made a Baronet (Freiherr). He continued his distinguished military career after the war, rising to the rank of lieutenant colonel, again being decorated, and moving to Austria to serve in the Austrian Emperor's elite corps of bodyguards. He married Johanna Freiin (Baroness) von Mayern. The youngest of their four children was Peter Zeno Freiherr von Pirquet, Clemens's father.

Peter Zeno Freiherr von Pirquet was well educated and politically active. He married Flora Freiin von Pereira-Arnstein of a distinguished Viennese family. Peter and Flora von Pirquet acquired a country estate not far from Vienna in Hirschstetten, and there Clemens was born on May 12, 1874, the sixth child and fourth son of the prosperous couple.[1] Clemens was shy as a young child, but nonetheless happy, and he had many boyhood friends in the village. Nursemaids helped Flora tend her large brood, and a tutor provided schooling for Clemens and his siblings. Flora, who was a devout Catholic, took special interest in the young Clemens. When the children grew older, the family moved to Vienna to take advantage of schools there. Flora von Pirquet enjoyed the social life of Vienna, and she was an accomplished hostess. Clemens entered the Schottengymnasium, a Benedictine school with a reputation for excellence that counted Johann Strauss, Jr., among its many distinguished alumni. Clemens was an apt student with special flares for both mathematics and music. After three years he transferred to a Jesuit boarding school in Kalksburg. There he excelled as a student, consistently achieving honors.

Clemens was singled out during his student days in Kalksburg as a good candidate for the priesthood, an idea that appealed greatly to his pious mother, who encouraged this career choice for her son. While entitled to be called Freiherr, he was one of the younger sons of the large family, and he did not expect to inherit the family land. A clerical life was pursued by many youths of such a family position at that time. Although urged to the priesthood by his mother, other members of his family were concerned about making such a decision at a young age. His father counseled him to study law, but that career did not appeal to him.

In 1892 Clemens von Pirquet entered the University of Innsbruck and began his studies of theology. A year later, he transferred to the University of Louvain in Belgium, where he earned a bachelor's degree in philosophy in 1894. During the spring of 1894 von Pirquet went with other students on a pilgrimage to Lourdes. That trip provided a time of profound introspection for the young student and appears to have solidified doubts in his mind. He decided to abandon his studies of theology and his career plans for the priesthood. To the disappointment of his family, he decided to study medicine, a field of endeavor not held in high social esteem in Austria at that time.

Doctor

Medical education in Europe in von Pirquet's time customarily included study at several medical schools with attendance at the courses offered by distinguished professors at each. Von Pirquet began his studies at the University of Vienna, which at that time had achieved prominence in pathology. After one year, he then moved to the University of Königsberg in East Prussia. Königsberg was a center of excellence in both surgery and physiology. Although von Pirquet did not excel as a student there, he acquired his first experience in experimentation at Königsberg; he was set to the task of studying the stability of electrodes being used in the physiology laboratory. Finally, von Pirquet returned to Austria to complete his medical studies at the University of Graz, where he earned academic honors and received his M.D. degree in 1900. Graz was the home of the famous professor of pediatrics Theodur Escherich, who is remembered today for having given his name to *Escherichia coli*, the bacterial denizen of the intestinal tract, but was notable in his time as one of the founders of academic pediatrics as a distinct medical discipline. Escherich regarded von Pirquet highly and encouraged him to become a pediatrician.

Following his graduation from medical school, von Pirquet went to Berlin for six months for additional studies in pediatrics. In Berlin he met Maria Christine van Heusen, a buxom and fun-loving young woman from Hanover with modern ideas, who was working in Berlin. Soon Clemens and Maria were in love and planning to be married. The von Pirquet family did not approve of this liaison, for they considered Maria van Heusen not to be of a social status appropriate for a young man of the Austrian nobility. Clemens was determined, however, and in 1904 the couple were married in Berlin. One of Clemens's brothers was the only von Pirquet family member in attendance at the wedding. The marriage was not without friction from the start and soon became problematic. Maria was barren as the result of complications of an earlier gynecologic procedure; the couple later adopted two children. Maria was a heavy smoker, and she became increasingly obese. She was querulous and an insomniac who spent much of the day in bed and took barbiturates every night. Frequently depressed, she made at least one unsuccessful attempt at suicide. An associate of von Pirquet reported that "although barely forty, she looked old, unkempt, and unattractive. Her speech was slurred from the effect of sleeping pills. Conversation was difficult. . . . "[2] Another visitor was somewhat kinder, although perhaps evasive, in his assessment: "She was very charming but an unusual and rather strange woman. She smoked excessively, even at that early date."[3] Maria was scorned by von Pirquet's friends, yet he remained faithful to her, not defending her but accepting and tolerating her difficult personality.

At the end of 1901, von Pirquet returned from Berlin to Vienna to undertake a two year internship and residency with Escherich, who had left Graz for more prestigious Vienna, at the Universitäts Kinderklinik of the St. Anna Children's Hospital. An exceptional group of trainees had assembled on Escherich's service in Vienna, notably including Franz Hamburger and Béla Schick; the latter became von Pirquet's close friend and associate. In 1903, von Pirquet became Escherich's clinical assistant. This appointment put him at the head of the pack of young Turks on Escherich's service and launched him upon his academic career.

Allergy

Clemens von Pirquet began his career at an exciting time in the medical world. Louis Pasteur had begun the scientific study of bacteria and Robert Koch had demonstrated convincingly that they caused human diseases. Edward Jenner had introduced vaccination for the prevention of smallpox, and Pasteur had successfully immunized against rabies. It was thus apparent that protective immunity could be induced against microbial diseases. In 1890 Emil von Behring, a disciple of Koch, discovered that he could transfer this immunity with serum, and within five years he was producing large amounts of horse antiserum to diphtheria toxin, with dramatic benefits to many. Von Pirquet became interested in this new field of medicine, and he undertook to study antibody-mediated reactions with Rudolf Kraus, a member of the medical faculty in Vienna and the discoverer of the precipitin reaction.

Von Pirquet was not happy in the laboratory environment, and he soon returned to devote his energies to the clinical arena. As Escherich's clinical assistant, Clemens von Pirquet found himself caring for patients on a ward for streptococcal disease. Paul Moser had developed an equine antiserum to streptococci and demonstrated that it agglutinated these bacteria. He had begun treating children with scarlet fever with this antiserum, giving doses as large as several hundred milliliters. Many of these children became ill following the administration of serum, and von Pirquet applied his quantitatively oriented mind to understanding their illness. He called the illness "serum disease," the forerunner of the modern designation "serum sickness." In collaboration with Béla Schick, his friend and junior colleague, he carefully plotted the time course of serum sickness, and from his observations he developed ideas that mark the beginning of the field of scientific endeavor we know today as immunology.

On April 2, 1903, von Pirquet deposited a remarkable letter with the Academy of Sciences in Vienna. Today, scientists with ideas for which they wish to insure their priority, but which are not yet sufficiently developed to justify a full manuscript in a scientific journal, send abstracts to and make presentations at scientific meetings or post their ideas on the Internet. In von Pirquet's time the accepted method of establishing one's place at the head of the scientific queue was by a letter of the type von Pirquet wrote. The text of this letter, to which he gave the title "On the Theory of Infectious Diseases," read:

> In many natural and experimentally induced diseases, the entry of the causative agent (infective or toxic) into the body, and the onset of symptoms, are separated by an interval of time known as the incubation period.
>
> These diseases and conditions, in the light of our present knowledge, offer so many analogous features that it is possible to regard them all from a common viewpoint.
>
> Their symptoms have a sudden onset, and consist of fever, general malaise (1–6) and exanthemata (1,4–6); are accompanied by a sudden drop in the leucocyte count—after a preliminary rise during the previous incubation period (4,6); and are followed by the appearance in the blood of antibodies which react specifically with the causative agent (1–3). These antibodies subsequently disappear, but for quite a long time afterwards the organism retains the capacity—on renewed contact with the causative agent—to repeat the whole process, in a shorter period (1–4).
>
> The conditions appertaining to these observations are:
>
> I)   Those following the subcutaneous injection of nonviable foreign substances of animal or bacterial origin:

a) Symptoms following the injection of foreign serum in man. (Observations in the Children's Hospital of St. Anna, publications on serum-therapy.) (1)
b) Symptoms following the injection of foreign serum into animals. (*v. Dungern; Hamburger and Moro*; and others.) (2) Under this heading can be included the symptoms following the injection of tuberculin.
II) Those following the introduction of viable bacteria with their metabolic products: Symptoms in horses associated with immunization with scarlatina streptococci. (3)
III) Those following the introduction of viable bacteria without their metabolic products:
a) Experimental conditions: Smallpox-vaccination. (Observations by *Bohn, Filatow and Sobotka,* and others; confirmed in the Children's Hospital of St. Anna.) (4)
b) Acute infectious diseases:
Variola (5)
Measles. (6)

From the above, I draw the following conclusions:
i) The length of the incubation period depends not only on the nature of the causative agent but also on that of the organism affected.
ii) The symptoms appear at the time the antibodies produced in the organism react with the causative agent.
iii) The lasting immunity thus acquired is due to the capacity of the organism to reproduce these antibodies more quickly—as shown by a shortening of the incubation period. There is a clinical difference between the immunity to toxins (group I) and to bacteria (group III) in that the reaction in the first case is stronger and in the second weaker according to the rapidity of its onset.

I shall be publishing in full the observations on which the foregoing conclusions are based, in conjunction with Dr. *Bela Schick*, within the next few months.

Vienna, April 2, 1903   sign. *Clemens v. Pirquet*[4]

The bracketed numbers von Pirquet included in the text of the third paragraph provided cross reference to items in the subsequent outline, with the bracketed numbers repeated at the end of the outline items.

Von Pirquet did not publish his ideas as promptly as his letter asserted he would, and the sealed document was not opened and read until five years later, when von Pirquet had become very confident in his hypotheses. While others had recognized antibodies, it was the young von Pirquet, scarcely through his formal training, who first grasped the pivotal concept that primary immunization is followed by accelerated anamnestic responses upon reinjection, the now-familiar-to-all "booster" response.

Let us consider the state of knowledge at the time that von Pirquet reached his conclusions. Jenner had used cow pox virus to immunize against smallpox. Pasteur had then taken a great step forward, and produced vaccines against bovine anthrax, swine erysipelas, and rabies. Emil von Behring had demonstrated that immunity to diphtheria toxin could be conveyed passively with horse antiserum, opening up a dramatic therapeutic modality that immediately stimulated many scientists to experiment with the administration of foreign sera to animals. Adverse reactions were soon recognized in animals, and von Behring noted them in some of his patients, calling them "paradoxical."[5] Von Pirquet called them "serum disease," anticipating the modern term "serum sickness," as noted above.

Paul Ehrlich, one of Koch's protégés and an expert chemist, had concluded that antigen-antibody reactions were stoichiometric ones analogous to simple chemical reactions. To explain the obvious differences between the reactions of cations with anions and antigens with antibodies, Ehrlich developed a complex "side chain" theory that allowed him to continue to think of these reactions as stoichiometric while accepting the variable combining ratios demonstrated by Kraus's precipitin reactions. Ehrlich received the Nobel Prize for this mistaken and now long-forgotten theory. Von Pirquet and Schick felt that Ehrlich's hypothesis did not explain accelerated and heightened reactions following reinjection (anamnestic responses) and that it was not tenable. We now know a great deal about the reaction of antibody with antigen. We recognize that Immunoglobulin-G is bivalent; immunoglobulin-M pentavalent. Antigens are variably multivalent. Precipitation is maximal at equivalence, and antibody-antigen complexes are soluble in antigen excess. In reading von Pirquet's hypotheses developed from his clinical observations, one cannot help but be impressed with his understanding of immunological reactions. He seems to have anticipated in a prescient, insightful way principles of immunochemistry that would not be developed for decades to come. The embryonic science of immunochemistry was beginning to manifest fetal movements; Clemens von Pirquet would attend its birth.

Beginning only two months after sending his sealed letter to the Academy of Sciences in Vienna, von Pirquet expressed his ideas in a series of letters to Professor Max Gruber in Munich, who had first demonstrated bacterial agglutination by antiserum. Gruber had challenged Ehrlich's ideas, feeling that physiological processes were too complex to be explained by the models of chemistry. In June of 1903 von Pirquet wrote to Gruber, "the basic fact from which I start is that, in serum sickness as well as in vaccination, the time from the first intoxication or infection until occurrence of the specific reaction is rather constant, while the incubation time is always shorter after revaccination or reinjection."[6] This is a very clear description of the anamnestic response, which had not been noted by previous observers. Gruber responded enthusiastically to von Pirquet, still at that time an unknown and very junior person, and the two men began a productive collaboration that shaped the young pediatrician's thinking and led him into the van of early twentieth-century immunology, a field that he largely created and molded. Von Pirquet's concept of toxin-antitoxin reactions, as revealed by a reading today of his correspondence with Gruber, anticipates modern immunochemical understanding of antigen-antibody reactions.

Today, physicians and their patients use the term allergy to describe such conditions as hay fever and angioneurotic edema. These entities were known in von Pirquet's time,[7] but the term allergy had not been applied to them. It was von Pirquet who coined the term in a short and now-famous paper entitled "Allergie" and published in 1906. It read, in part:

> The connection between immunity and hypersensitivity appears to me most evident from experience with vaccination for smallpox. A recently revaccinated individual appears to be hypersensitive when compared with one vaccinated for the first time because he reacts much more quickly to the infection. At the same time he is protected, for the vaccinial process is characterized by an insignificant local reaction and all constitutional signs are absent.

Immunity and hypersensitivity can thus be closely related but the words contradict one another; their combination is very strained. The concept of immunity is carried over from the time when hypersensitivity was not known. . . . We need a new, more general term, devoid of bias, to denote the change experienced by an organism from its contact with an organic poison, whether live or inanimate. The reaction toward a given toxin of an individual who has not previously been in contact with it differs from the reaction of an individual who has. Such a changed reaction is shown by a vaccinated individual toward calf lymph, by the syphilitic toward the syphilis virus, by the tuberculous toward tuberculin, and by the individual injected with horse serum toward horse serum. The treated individual is far from being insensitive. All that can be said is that his ability to react has changed.

For this general concept of a change in ability to react, I suggest the term *allergy*. Allos means "other" and hence a deviation from the original state or from normal behavior, as in allorhythmia and allotropism.

The vaccinated, the tuberculous, and the individual injected with horse serum become allergic toward the respective foreign body. On the other hand, a foreign substance which induces the organism to react in a changed manner to its single or repeated introduction into the body is an *allergen*. The word is modeled on the term antigen (Detre-Deutsch) in a manner highly discordant with the laws of philology. An antigen is a substance which is capable of producing antibodies; the concept of an allergen includes, in addition to the antigens, numerous protein substances which do not promote formation of antibodies but cause hypersensitivity. . . . All organisms causing infectious diseases which are followed by immunity are allergens; so are the toxins of mosquitoes and of bees, since they induce manifestations of hypo- or hypersensitivity. For the same reason, we can include the pollen causing hay fever (Wolff-Eisner), the urticaria-producing substances of strawberries and of crustaceans, and probably also a series of organic substances giving rise to idiosyncrasy.

The term immunity should be limited to those states in which the introduction of a foreign substance does not result in any clinical reaction. Thus there exists a complete absence of sensitivity, which may be conditioned by natural immunity (alexins), by antitoxins (active or passive immunity, as against diphtheria or tetanus), or by some kind of adaptation to the toxin (Wassermann and Citron).[8]

Von Pirquet meant the term *allergy* to include not only hay fever from pollens and hives from strawberries but also all hypersensitivity reactions. He clearly noted the differences between immunity and hypersensitivity, assigning the latter to his newly defined *allergy*. Finally, he coined and defined the term *allergen*, which is still used today, albeit with a somewhat altered meaning.

In 1911 von Pirquet published in the *Archives of Internal Medicine* a remarkable scholarly, state-of-the-art, comprehensive review paper entitled "Allergy," in which he reviewed the existing knowledge of immune responses in infectious diseases and also set forth his views on allergy, as he defined it, in clear detail. Referring to reactions to horse serum, he wrote the following elegant description of serum sickness:

The first injection of horse-serum which we use as a carrier of antitoxin in diphtheria, tetanus, scarlet fever and epidemic meningitis has not only an antitoxic influence, but often causes symptoms of its own, which consist in urticaria fever, edema and pains in the joints. They are due to the horse-serum, for they show themselves also after injection of the serum of healthy horses not previously treated with diphtheria or other toxins (Bokay, Johannessen).

These symptoms to which Schick and I have given the name of "serum disease" occur only occasionally immediately after the injection. There is nearly always an incubation time of eight to twelve days up to the outbreak of the symptoms. On a repetition of the injection a different behavior is noted [as illustrated by the following clinical history].

E.E.; injection of 200 c.c. scarlatina serum of Moser. On the evening of the seventh day a severe serum disease set in, which consisted in a swelling of the regionary lymph-glands, fever up to 40.5, edema and rash, the latter first consisting of urticaria; later on it had the character of erythema multiforme (Marfan's *érythème marginé aberrant*). Thirty-eight days later fifteen children received immunizing doses of 1 c.c. antidiphtheritic serum, among them E.E., who showed after eight hours, fever and a swelling of the skin of the lower arm on the point of injection. The next morning a diffuse red, painful swelling up to the middle of the upper arm was noticed, and in the afternoon a general rash of urticaria character. The fever lasted thirty-six hours, then the swelling decreased gradually. On the sixth day after this injection, again a general rash.

We shall study in these cases the properties of allergy against horse-serum in man.

1. Allergy According to Time.— The symptoms after the first injec-

tion of E.E. appeared on the seventh day; after reinjection, after eight hours.

2. Quantitative Allergy.— Of the fifteen children who were injected at the same time with E.E., 10 had not received the serum previously. Only one of them showed a very slight swelling at the same time that E.E. showed his severe symptoms. Between the sixth and eighth day, slight general symptoms were noticed in four of them.

The severe reaction which E.E. showed was, therefore, not due to a property of the horse-serum which was used in this second injection, but was due to a subjective disposition. He was extremely hypersensitive, and this hypersensitiveness was an acquired one, for he had not reacted in that way after the first injection.

3. Qualitative Allergy.— After the first injection there were no local reactions on the point of injection, but general symptoms, such as fever, urticaria and hydrops. The second injection provoked an intense redness and swelling at the point of inoculation. In other cases the reinjection is followed by general phenomena of short duration, which are sometimes accompanied by collapse. This collapse is never seen in serum disease occurring after a normal incubation time.[9]

Here it is evident that von Pirquet's concepts included not only altered reactions and anamnestic responses but also specificity as characteristic of allergic reactions. The local reactions he described are clearly those of the type first described in 1903 by Maurice Arthus, which now are commonly known by that scientist's name.

The Tuberculin Test

As was noted in Chapter 5, Robert Koch had noted that tuberculous individuals reacted to the injection of his tuberculin, which his clinical colleagues had administered to them as a therapy for the disease. Soon, veterinarians observed that cattle reacting to tuberculin invariably had lesions of tuberculosis when slaughtered, and physicians began using the systemic reactions to injected tuberculin as an aid to the diagnosis of tuberculosis. Von Pirquet reasoned that the intracutaneous method in use for smallpox vaccination could be used for tuberculin testing. In 1909 he read a paper to the Berlin Medical Society proposing that the reaction observed on the second day following intracutaneous inoculation of tuberculin could be used to diagnose tuberculous infection.[10] Shortly thereafter, he described his technique in an article published in the *Journal of the American Medical Association*:

> My method of applying the test is as follows: The skin of the forearm is scrubbed with ether; then two drops of undiluted old tuberculin are dropped about four inches distant from each other. Then, with a vaccinating lancet, the point of which has the form of a small chisel, a superficial circular scarification is made between the two drops (for the control of the traumatic redness following the small scarification). Finally, the same scarification is made inside of the two drops. . . . The papula is examined after twenty-four and forty-eight hours. It is considered positive when the tuberculin scarifications are clearly different from the control places, but the inflammatory reactive area must measure at least 1/6 of an inch (5 mm.).[11]

It remained only for Charles Mantoux to introduce the technique of injecting intracutaneously measured amounts of tuberculin with a syringe and fine cannulated needle in 1908 and for Florence Seibert to prepare tuberculin purified protein derivative (PPD) in the 1930s for medicine to arrive at the technique currently accepted as the gold standard for the diagnosis of tuberculous infection.

Clemens von Pirquet did more than simply describe the technique of tuberculin testing. He recognized the importance and utility of tuberculin reactions. "Only those individuals who have already been infected with tuberculosis show an inflammatory reaction at the point of vaccination," he wrote, "whereas the healthy individuals show no reaction at all."[12] He went on to study tuberculin reactivity in Viennese children of varying ages with or without manifest tuberculosis, concluding that "in the first two years [of life] . . . an infection practically does not occur without the existence of some clinical phenomena. . . . In older children the presence of a tuberculin reactivity may be compatible with apparently perfect health."[13] The data upon which he based this conclusion, now well established as fact, are presented in Figure 7.1, taken from his paper. He further noted that in the adolescent and post-adolescent years, girls were more susceptible than boys to tuberculosis. His observations anticipated by three decades many of those made by Wade Hampton

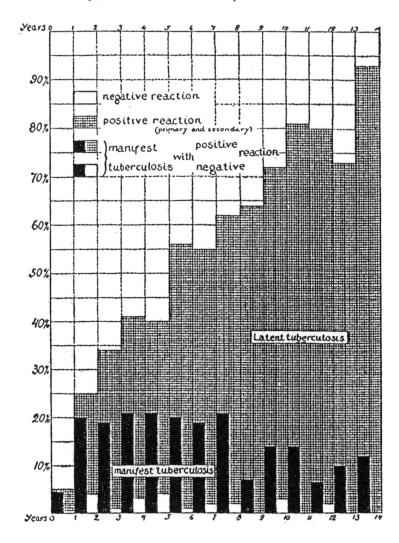

Figure 7.1. Tuberculin reactivity as the percent of individuals reacting positively plotted against age in years by Clemens von Pirquet for 1,407 children tested at Escherich's pediatric clinic in Vienna. Although the reactor rate reached more than 90% by age 14, this should not be taken to reflect the reactor rate for children in Vienna as a whole, for children referred to Escherich's clinic were a biased sample, reflecting the interest of von Pirquet and others at the clinic in tuberculosis. From Von Pirquet C. The frequency of tuberculosis in children. JAMA 1909; 675–8. Copyrighted 1909, American Medical Association. Figure reproduced with permission.

Frost (Chapter 8) and his colleagues in their much more extensive studies of the natural history of tuberculous infection in Tennessee.

With a reliable means of diagnosing tuberculous infection at hand, von Pirquet was able to study the natural history of this infection in the children whom he saw, and he contributed enormously to our understanding of host-parasite relationships in tuberculosis. "I regard this reaction of importance," he wrote of the tuberculin test, "in so far as it may enable us to recognize the initial stages of tuberculosis."[14] In 1909 he expanded on the pioneering observations described above and provided an insightful discussion that has rarely been equalled since:

> The first form of tuberculosis in infants . . . is very often mistakenly looked upon as a gastrointestinal marasmus. Without showing any signs on the outside of the body, the children gradually lose in weight and die after a few months. In the post mortem examination you will find a tuberculous condition and caseation of nearly all the glands of the lungs, of the peritoneum and mesentery. . . . Sometimes the post mortem examination shows besides this, tuberculous knots in the brain, bones, spleen, liver, and kidneys. The second form resembles more the tuberculosis in adults. . . . In the post mortem examination one finds, besides a tuberculosis of the bronchial glands, a lobular pneumonia of tuberculous character, very often combined with cavities. A third form comprises the cases of caseous pneumonia. . . . The last form, which is more common than the others, is miliary tuberculosis. . . . Among the symptoms of the miliary form, the brain affection, tuberculous meningitis, nearly always predominates. . . .
>
> There is a great difference between the consequences of tuberculous infection in infancy, especially of the first year, and the later stages of childhood. We now know that a large number of children between the ages of six and fourteen are infected with tuberculosis without showing any clinical symptoms. In cases of this kind, tuberculosis is localized in the lymph nodes and does not spread over the whole body. In infancy the power of localization of tuberculosis does not yet seem to be developed.[15]

In the same paper, von Pirquet noted that tuberculin reactivity took "some weeks after the infection" to appear, that it waned with the passing of years, and that tuberculin reactions were often negative in children with measles. For the lack of reactivity in measles he coined the term anergy, a word still in general use. Anergy, he also noted, occurred in patients with disseminated or miliary tuberculosis, in cachectic patients, in patients with lepromatous leprosy, and "some few cases . . . [for which] none of the former explanations can be applied." These statements remain true to this day, and the phenomena von Pirquet discovered are being rediscovered today and discussed by modern investigators. In order to deal with waning of reactivity he recommended, "All children are submitted to the cutaneous test. The following day they are inspected. . . . A week later those who showed no reaction are again tested. . . . "[16] Modern health workers interested in tuberculosis control will recognize in this recommendation the currently popular dual-test technique used to avoid confusion introduced by the booster phenomenon.

During this period of enormous productivity, which spanned no more than a half dozen years, von Pirquet often worked in collaboration Béla Schick, his former student. The two of them unravelled the mysteries of serum sickness, and von Pirquet's concepts of this condition gave birth to fundamental concepts of the modern field of immunology. With respect to childhood tuberculosis, von Pirquet's clinical observations were again trail-blazing. Clemens von Pirquet's contemporaries recognized the importance of his work, and his reputation grew rapidly. He was invited to speak at international fora both in Europe and North America. Doctors came to Vienna to meet him and learn from him. He charmed these visitors, who found him to be handsome as well as friendly and hospitable, sometimes taking them on walks in the Austrian Alps, always impressing them with his energy and knowledge. He was on the way to becoming the preeminent pediatrician of his time.

Distinguished Professor

Although some of the papers cited above had not yet been published, Clemens von Pirquet, now 34 years old, entered the year 1908 confident of his ideas and increasingly recognized for his achievements. Early in that year he asked that his sealed letter to the Austrian Academy of Sciences be opened and read, thus cementing his claim to priority for his work. Moreover, he had developed into a charming and brilliant lecturer, fluent in several languages. The world of academic biomedical science was about to knock at his door.

Émile Roux had succeeded Louis Pasteur as director of the Pasteur Institute, and he sought to add von Pirquet to the list of distinguished investigators interested in host responses to infection at that prestigious institute. The young pediatrician was flattered by the offer and gave it serious thought, meanwhile continuing what had by then become an almost continual round of presentations. After he had given a lecture in Paris on his tuberculin test, he was introduced by Robert Koch to William Welch, the distinguished pathologist and dean of Johns Hopkins School of Medicine, who was travelling in Europe. Welch was impressed with the young pediatrician. He also consulted Escherich, who endorsed his former student. Von Pirquet had been invited to participate in an international congress on tuberculosis to be held that year in Washington, DC, and Welch asked him to visit Johns Hopkins while he was in the United States and consider an appointment there. Putting off a reply to Roux and the Pasteur Institute, von Pirquet agreed to consider an offer from Johns Hopkins.

Johns Hopkins was an unmarried Baltimore business man and philanthropist who gave his entire fortune to found both a university and a hospital in Baltimore. The terms of his endowment linked the two together and provided for establishing a school of medicine at the university. Johns Hopkins University opened in 1876; the hospital, construction of which was delayed by the poor performance of some investments in Johns Hopkins's estate, in 1889; the medical school in 1893. It was largely due to the vision of John Shaw Billings, who first served as a consultant to the nascent hospital and then became a member of its board of directors, that Johns Hopkins Hospital and Medical School were planned as institutions not only of medical care and medical education but also of medical research. No other medical school in North America had its roots so firmly planted in the fertile soil of clinical research as did this new institution. Among the first faculty members recruited to Johns Hopkins was the New York pathologist William Welch, who had recently established North America's first experimental pathology laboratory at Bellevue Hospital. Welch, who soon became dean of the new medical school, added an additional innovative element—

the organization of the hospital into departments. He also began at Johns Hopkins the practice of recruiting faculty on a full-time, salaried basis, a costly system about which he had some personal doubts.

Clemens von Pirquet presented his paper on the tuberculin test to the Sixth International Congress on Tuberculosis in Washington on September 28, 1908. He then visited Baltimore where Welch hosted a dinner for him at the Maryland Club, a dinner at which Johns Hopkins professors could evaluate the young candidate. At that time, plans were being drawn for the Harriet Lane Home, a new children's hospital at Johns Hopkins, the endowment for which had been provided in the estate of Harriet Lane Johnston, who had lost two sons to childhood illnesses. Von Pirquet would have an opportunity to influence the plans for this facility at which his new Department of Pediatrics would be based. Welch and his colleagues were favorably impressed with von Pirquet, and the following January the trustees of the university offered him the chair of the newly created department. His salary would be $4,000 per year, with the opportunity to earn additional income in clinical practice. Von Pirquet accepted the offer.

Clemens and Maria von Pirquet arrived in Baltimore in February 1909. They were well received by the faculty of Johns Hopkins and quickly made friends in the university community. They purchased a large house, and Maria established what one contemporary called "a veritable ménage which his salary could not support."[17] Clemens threw himself with vigor into the business of establishing a new department and building a new hospital. He was described by a colleague as "A fascinating speaker. . . . A brilliant scientist. A first class executive."[18]

The move to Baltimore marked a watershed in the life and career of Clemens von Pirquet. Never again would he make contributions to medical science of the importance of those made earlier in his career. Never again would he turn his mind to the field of immunology. He continued to present the observations he had made in Vienna and to publish scientific articles. Indeed, some of the studies of the natural history of tuberculosis considered above were published from Johns Hopkins, although they were based on earlier work. In April following his arrival at Johns Hopkins he delivered the annual oration of the faculty, addressing the topic of infectious diseases. After considering at length the necessity and value of isolating children with communicable diseases, he turned to the teaching of infectious diseases. "Only a special training in infectious diseases hospitals," he argued, "can give the teacher sufficient experience to instruct the student properly."[19] This theme would recur later after his return to the Kinderklinik of Vienna.

Probably motivated largely by financial difficulties—a profitable pediatric consultation practice had not emerged to augment his salary—von Pirquet decided to leave Johns Hopkins when he was offered an appointment in Breslau, Germany (now Wroclaw, Poland) scarcely more than a year after his arrival. He may also have been influenced by dissatisfaction with a life that so frequently revolved around the details of constructing a new hospital rather than practicing medicine. His letter of resignation to the president of the university is of interest, because it clearly was intended not to close the door on Johns Hopkins too tightly and also, perhaps, to distance himself from the administrative chores of planning a new hospital building, should he return:

March 6th, 1910

Dear President Remsen,

Upon nomination by the Medical Faculty of the University of Breslau, the Prussian ministry of education has offered me the position of professor of pediatrics at that University.

I have accepted this call.

Mr. Blanchard Randall has suggested that I should not offer my resignation here but that I should ask for a leave of absence and have a chance to consider the question again after having tried the position in Breslau.

Mr. Randall's suggestion was very agreeable to me, as it gives me the possibility of coming back and continuing and developing the work here under more favorable conditions for both of us.

It would be gratifying to me if some such arrangement could be made by which my relations with the Johns Hopkins University and Hospital were not completely severed at this time, so that I might assume the position in Breslau and still might have the opportunity, if on trial of this position it seemed to me best to return here, to be able to do so. Of course my salary would cease during my absence from the first of May, and I should agree to communicate at least before the first of next January to you my final decision, it being understood that the University is at [the] same time free to fill my chair if it so desires. If I return to this University I shall on January the first 1911 request an additional leave of absence until the Harriet Lane Home is completed.

Very respectfully ours,

(signed) Clemens Freiherr von Pirquet[20]

On behalf of the university, Remsen promptly acceded to von Pirquet's request for a leave of absence. The following January, although von Pirquet had not followed through with the further communication promised in his resignation letter, President Remsen tried to induce him to return with an offer of a truly full-time appointment with "a yearly salary of $7,500 on condition that you devote yourself entirely to the care of hospital patients (both free and pay), teaching and investigation, and do not engage in private practice. . . . " "In order to make possible the payment of so large a salary, which will be the largest thus paid to any professor in the University," he wrote, "you and your assistants will be expected to supervise the treatment of all private patients admitted to the Children's Hospital with the understanding that whatever fees are paid for such services will go into the Treasury of the Hospital and not to you."[21] The offer also held out the hope of establishing a new salary scale for full-time department heads of $10,000 annually at some unspecified future date. Several junior faculty members at Johns Hopkins came forward with an offer to Remsen to provide the $2,500 necessary to increase this offer to $10,000 immediately, an extraordinary proposal, which Remsen did not accept. Von Pirquet did not reply, and in May 1911, Remsen wrote to him asking for a reply by cable. Finally, on June 27, von Pirquet replied. His letter stated that he "did not consider a yearly salary of $7,500 an adequate remuneration." He would have accepted $10,000, he indicated, but the matter was now closed as he had agreed to leave Breslau and return to Vienna.[22]

Theodur Escherich, von Pirquet's mentor and beloved professor, died suddenly in 1911. A new pediatric hospital to replace the St. Anna's Children's Hospital, where the young von Pirquet had served as an intern and resident, was nearing completion at the time, and Escherich would have been its director. Without hesitation, the University of Vienna turned to Clemens von Pirquet and, equally unhesitatingly, he accepted the call. The new Kinderklinik was dedicated to the memory of Escherich on November 13, 1911. Von Pirquet gave the opening lecture, speaking as he had at Johns Hopkins about the teaching of infectious diseases.

Except for a brief few weeks in 1924 at the University of Minnesota, an interlude reminiscent of the Baltimore year, Clemens von Pirquet spent the rest of his life at the Kinderklinik. Richard Wagner, his principal associate for many years at the Kinderklinik and his biographer, devotes half of his book to the seventeen years he spent there. Yet, considered with reference to von Pirquet's earlier contributions to medical science, these were nonproductive years occupied in clinical practice and the pursuit of unattainable or unimportant goals. At the same time, his clinical reputation was unsurpassed, and his daily ward rounds were crowded with visitors from across the globe.

World War I had a profound effect on von Pirquet's life. Surely an internationalist, von Pirquet was also a patriotic Austrian who defended strongly Austria's declaration of war on Serbia after the assassination of Archduke Ferdinand. As Austria mobilized for war, the Kinderklinik was left with only three physicians, all too old for military service: von Pirquet, Schick, and a Russian emigré. These three men carried the entire patient-care load, leaving little time for research. Moreover, the war isolated Austria, and news of medical advances did not reach Vienna during the war years.

Nutrition, Anthropometrics, and Vital Statistics

Following his arrival at the Kinderklinik in Vienna, von Pirquet turned his attention to aspects of childhood development. He felt that calories were a poor way to measure the nutritional value of food. Coal, he pointed out, has caloric value but no nutritional value. Milk, he argued, would make a relevant standard of nutrition, and he proposed a system based on the nutritional equivalent of milk. The basic unit, a nem, was the nutritional value of one milliliter of milk. Many found this system to be cumbersome and difficult to work with, but in a tribute following von Pirquet's death it was defended by the eminent British nutritionist Harriette Chick:

Theoretical objections can be brought against Pirquet's "Nem" system, as for example, in the rejection of the calorie as a measure of nutritive value for a new arbitrary unit—viz., the "nem" or food valued of 1 c.cm. milk (0.67 calorie). No one, however, who has seen the "Nem" system in working, can deny its success in practice. For in this system the nutritional value of foods is assessed against a *standard which can be seen and handled.* In the kitchens, where the nursing staff received an important part of their training, the working unit, 100 nems or 1 hectonem, is visualised as 100 c.cm. of milk, seen in the graduated cylinders which function as the ordinary kitchen measures. The newest probationer soon realises that the addition of 8 g. of sugar or cereal in the preparation of an infant's food increases the food value of the meal by 50 per cent.[23]

With the end of World War I, the victorious allies created a commission headed by Herbert Hoover to provide emergency relief for the civilian populations of Germany and Austria. Hoover named von Pirquet commissioner General for Austria, and in this capacity the pediatrician was charged with the equitable distribution of food to the population. Von Pirquet applied his nem system to assigning appropriate rations. However, nems did not spread beyond Austria and these units failed to replace conventional calories.

Today pediatricians and parents follow the growth and development of infants and children by plotting their height, weight, and head size against curves developed for normal children. Those curves had not yet been developed in von Pirquet's day, but he realized the importance of tracking childhood growth. He developed elaborate tables of normal measurements that were forerunners of the later graphs of these curves, but he went far beyond those measurements in a manner that appears abnormally obsessive to the modern reader. For example, he developed a table relating sitting height to the cube root of the weight of the heart and to pulse rate for both boys and girls and devised mathematical formulas to express the relationships of these parameters.[24]

Von Pirquet's colleague, friend, and biographer, Richard Wagner, described his last few years as his most creative period. In fact, von Pirquet was becoming increasingly obsessed with numbers and, in Wagner's words, "His mind indulged in abstractions and he was fascinated by numbers and graphic analyses. . . . It was no longer *what* he conceived of that was of importance to him, but the *way* in which it was expressed and exhibited."[25] His devotion to clinical medicine was pushed aside by a new devotion to ciphers. Wagner described him at that time as "schizothymic;" schizoaffective might be a better, more modern term.

Von Pirquet devoted himself to an extensive analysis of vital statistics from England and Wales, and concluded that fatal disease had a "center of gravity." He developed elaborate mathematical formulas for determining the days upon which certain diseases were most likely to occur. In fact, he was observing the well-known seasonal incidence of many infectious diseases. In 1927 he published an elaborate, perhaps bizarre chart consisting of overlapping ovoids superimposed on a circular calendar—a venn diagram on an Aztec calendar![26] He also developed graphs demonstrating that different diseases had different ages of peak mortality. With this preoccupation with numerical data, no new concepts of enduring value emerged from his once-productive, now-obsessed mind.

On February 28, 1929, in a double suicide, Clemens Freiherr von Pirquet and his wife Maria ended their lives with potassium cyanide. Unproductive and perhaps tormented by a disturbed and obsessed mind in his last decade, Clemens von Pirquet whimpered to the tragic end of his life. But what a bang he made early in his career. He described serum sickness and anamnestic responses. He devised the tuberculin skin test, which to this day remains the gold standard for the diagnosis of tuberculous infection. He elucidated the natural history of childhood tuberculosis. He coined the terms *allergy*, *allergen*, and *anergy*. More than any other, he was the pioneer who founded the science of immunology.

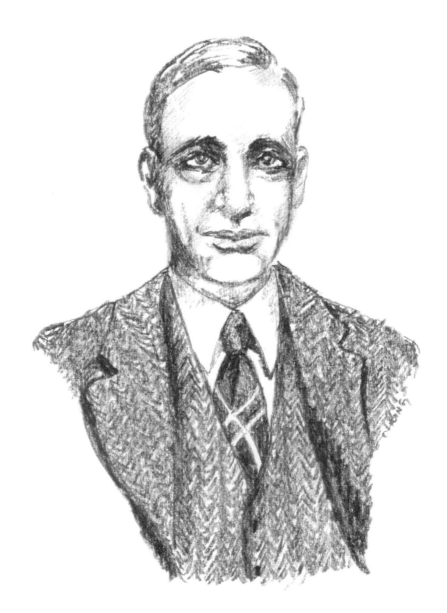

Wade Hampton Frost

Wade Hampton Frost
1880–1938
Pioneer of Epidemiology

As one travels through Fauquier County, Virginia, today, with the huge urban metroplex of America's capital to the east and the ancient scarps of the Appalachian mountains to the west, one is surrounded by lush and gentle countryside. Green grass carpets rolling meadows, and fences confine horses and cattle to verdant pastures. The land is fertile, and an aura of tranquility pervades every farm, hamlet, and town. Here sits Marshall, one block wide, the village in which Wade Hampton Frost entered the world on March 30, 1880.[1]

Turn-of-the-Century Virginia
and the Making of a Doctor

Fifteen years after the end of the Civil War, Frost was born into a rural Virginia that was undergoing political and social change but that largely escaped the tumultuous reconstruction that enveloped much of the South. Virginia had backed reluctantly into the Civil War, one of the last states to secede, yet had become a major battleground. Marshall is only about fifteen miles west of the battlefield of Manassas. The agricultural economy of this part of Virginia was more diversified than that of the great plantations to the south, and it better survived the transformation from slave labor to contract workers and share-cropping. Still, those postwar years were not prosperous times in Virginia. Political activity during Frost's boyhood years was in transition and decline. Democrats followed Republicans, who had taken over the state immediately after the war, and the state's constitution was rewritten to disenfranchise not only former slaves and their children but all persons lacking in education and wealth. Aristocracy, not democracy, defined Virginia politics of the times. The dominant popular political mood was one of apathy, however, and the numbers of voters participating in elections declined dramatically, reaching its nadir about 1910.[2]

Frost came from a long line of physicians. His great, great grandfather, Christopher Frost, was a surgeon in Norfolk, England. His grandfather, Thomas Frost, was a physician in colonial Charleston, South Carolina, where he served on the faculty of the Medical College of Charleston. His father, Henry Frost, also a physician, had joined the Confederate army as an assistant surgeon during the Civil War, and following the war he left the family home in Charleston to settle in Marshall, Virginia. There he established a medical practice and joined the Fauquier Medical Society, becoming its president in 1889.[3] Wade Hampton Frost was born into a family belonging to Virginia's gentry and a family with long traditions in medicine and public service.

Medicine at the end of the nineteenth century had entered a period of rapid gains in knowledge of the pathogenesis of disease, sparked by the work of European medical scientists. Laennec and Virchow had established the anatomic basis for diseases, Pasteur and Koch the importance of microorganisms as pathogenic infectious agents, and von Behring the role of antiserum therapy. Medical practice in Virginia did not lag far behind that in Europe; the journals of medical societies reported the discoveries made in Europe, and American pharmaceutical firms took up the production of therapeutic agents. Quinine and phenacetin were mainstays of every physician's black bag.

Doctor Henry Frost and his wife, Sabra J. Walker, raised eight children, of whom Wade Hampton Frost was the seventh. The boy was named for a Confederate general, whom Henry Frost much admired. A family story repeatedly recounted by Frost's daughter relates that Henry Frost's mind wandered during the baptism of his seventh child. When asked by the clergyman, "How shall this child be called?" the daydreaming father could not remember the chosen name. "Wade Hampton," he blurted out, for his reverie of the moment was focused on the Civil War general under whom he had served.

A quiet lad and an avid reader, Frost's early education was provided entirely at home by his outgoing and energetic mother. At an early age, he evinced an interest in medicine, and he accompanied his father on his rounds as he cared for his rural Virginia patients. At age fifteen the young Frost enrolled in a military academy in Danville, Virginia, where he studied for one year. The following year he spent at Randolph Macon Academy. Thereafter he worked for a year as a clerk in a local store.

In 1898, now eighteen years old, Frost entered the University of Virginia where he pursued a liberal arts education and was active in fraternity life and extracurricular activities. One can assume that his campus life included a good measure of frivolity, for these were the "gay nineties." Three years later he received the Bachelor of Arts degree and entered the medical school for a two-year course of study. Graduating in 1903 with the MD degree, he had received a reasonably strong didactic orientation to medicine, but little clinical experience. The University of Virginia was founded by Thomas Jefferson, and the teaching of medical sciences was included from its inception. However, from Jefferson's time, the emphasis in the curriculum was on the scientific basis of medicine and not on its practical aspects. To gain clinical experience, Frost followed the example of many of Virginia's medical graduates and went to New York City, where he "rode the ambulance" as a substitute intern at Bellevue Hospital and at St. John's Hospital in Yonkers. A year later he returned to Virginia to spend a year as an intern at St. Vincent's Hospital in Norfolk. By contemporaneous standards this course of medical education was a rigorous one, and his two years of internships provided him with more clinical experience than was had by most young doctors embarking upon their professional careers at that time. Wade Hampton Frost had become a competent physician and clinician.

The Public Health Service

Perhaps stimulated by the promise of intellectual challenge, perhaps motivated by his family's history of government service, or perhaps simply following a path well trodden by a large number of his fellow medical graduates of the University of Virginia, Frost took the qualifying examinations for a commission in the United States Public Health and Marine Hospital Service. He passed the examinations, received his commission, and in February of 1905 reported for duty as an Assistant Surgeon at the Marine Hospital in Baltimore, Maryland. The United States Public Health and Marine Hospital Service had been established in 1798 by an act of the Fifth United States Congress to provide for "the temporary relief and maintenance of sick or disabled seamen in the hospitals or other proper institutions now established in the several ports of the United States."[4] Funds to defray the cost were collected by levying a charge of twenty cents per month against the wages of all American seamen. The service attracted talented physicians, many of them graduates of the University of Virginia, and the Public Health Service Hygienic Laboratory in Washington became a center of investigation of infectious diseases. Twenty-five years later, in 1930, that laboratory became the major component of the newly created National Institute of Health of the United States Public Health Service. Frost, who had spent much of his early career at the laboratory and was by then a distinguished professor of epidemiology, was appointed to its board.

Within a few months of his enlistment in the Public Health Service, Frost's life was changed forever when he was assigned to a team attempting to deal with an epidemic of yellow fever in New Orleans. During the preceding four years, Walter Reed, William Gorgas, and others in Cuba and Panama had established that this often-fatal viral infection was transmitted by mosquitos and that mosquito control would bring with it control of yellow fever. The team that Frost joined was attempting to apply this new information in the face of an epidemic. This exciting assignment was Frost's introduction to epidemiologic field work— to what is often called "shoe leather" epidemiology. Frost and his coworkers diligently pursued the deadly insects, eliminating their breeding places, and for the first time in history a yellow fever epidemic was aborted before winter temperatures stopped the breeding of mosquitos. In fact, following this public health campaign, mosquito-control programs were rapidly instituted elsewhere in the United States, and there have been no significant yellow fever outbreaks in North America since.

Frost spent the next two years assigned as a medical officer to the Revenue Cutter Service, now the United States Coast Guard, which then and now drew its medical officers from the Public Health Service. He served at a training school for cadets in Curtis Bay, Maryland. This assignment meant summer cruises on Coast Guard vessels, and Frost's horizons widened at that time as he visited European, African, and

Caribbean ports. Assignments of this type were usual ones for Public Health Service Officers, but Frost was destined to break loose from this mold, and in the fall of 1908 he was sent to the Public Health Service Hygienic Laboratory in Washington, which, as noted, was the forerunner of the present National Institutes of Health. He was assigned to work on waterborne typhoid fever, a major health problem in Washington and other American cities at the time.

While many of his initial laboratory duties were fairly routine and devoted to the monitoring of drinking water supplies for Washington, he was soon caught up in the excitement of microbiologic investigation and the discipline it demanded. He published two papers describing an organism he isolated from Washington tap water.[5] He translated the need for sound data in studies conducted at the laboratory bench to a similar need for rigorous data in field investigations. Within a year he was promoted and placed in charge of a field study of an epidemic of typhoid in Williamson, West Virginia. John Snow, who lived in London during the nineteenth century and whom Frost came to admire greatly, had demonstrated in 1849 that cholera was waterborne and in 1854 identified the Broad Street pump as the source of an outbreak of this disease. Two years later William Budd demonstrated that typhoid could also be a waterborne infection. These two great English epidemiologists had made the fundamental observations that these bacterial diseases were transmitted through contaminated water, thus setting the course for Frost as he journeyed to Williamson.

In an investigation reminiscent of the earlier effort of Hermann Biggs in Plymouth, Pennsylvania (Chapter 6), Frost first turned his attention to sewage and water systems in the town. Williamson, he wrote in his report, "is at present only partially provided with a closed sewer system, consisting of a forty-one inch brick main, and smaller branch sewers of tiling. This system, constructed in 1907, . . . terminates in an open ravine about one hundred yards distant from the river, and through this ravine empties into the Tug River about opposite . . . the intake for the water supply."[6] Noting that water supplied to the town from the river was inadequately purified, Frost commented, "the water supplied is of very displeasing appearance. . . . It is frequently too black to be fit for bathing and laundry purposes, and often has an offensive odor. . . . Owing to the dangerous and unpleasant character of the city water supply, a considerable portion of the population of Williamson use[s] other water for drinking purposes."[7]

Having thus set the stage for his investigation, Frost then turned to the typhoid epidemic itself. No records were available, but conversations with local physicians made it evident that typhoid had not been recognized as a major health problem in the Williamson for at least a decade. Then, within three months, 152 cases occurred, representing one in every thirty-three residents. Frost carefully mapped the town and plotted the cases. He graphed the time course of the epidemic. He investigated dairies and other food sources. He surveyed the sanitation and water systems of Williamson, collected clinical and epidemiologic data on all of the incident typhoid cases, and he surveyed the incidence of diarrheal disease in the town. The amount of work accomplished by Frost, working essentially alone over a three-week period, was prodigious. In the end, he concluded that the epidemic probably began with fecal contamination of the water supply and was then sustained by close household contact until it ran its course. Finally, he made recommendations concerning water purification, sewage disposal, supervision of food supplies, and the care of patients. This masterful study marked the debut of Frost as an exceptionally talented field epidemiologist.

Frost undertook similar investigations of epidemics of typhoid fever in Arkansas and Iowa and of an outbreak of what was probably streptococcal pharyngitis in Baltimore. Then, in 1913, the Public Health Service established a laboratory at an abandoned Marine Hospital in the riverside city of Cincinnati, Ohio to study water pollution, and Frost was named its director, a position for which he was well qualified both by experience and temperament. Focusing on fecal contamination of drinking water supplies and on such waterborne diseases as typhoid fever and cholera, Frost noted that only eleven percent of sewage discharged into the Ohio River was treated in any manner,[8] and that nationwide no more than ten to fifteen percent of sewage was treated.[9] Frost's studies of waterborne diseases, beginning in Williamson and culminating in Cincinnati, are important to view not simply as epidemiologic investigations but as molding experiences during which he became fascinated with the quantitation of epidemiologic data. This mathematical way of thinking was to dominate much of his career and become one of his great contributions to medical science.

Frost's years in Cincinnati were not entirely devoted to the laboratory. Susan Haxall—from a well-established Richmond family with a summer home in Middleburg, Virginia, just north of Marshall, and whom Frost had courted in Washington where she was teaching dance during the time he was stationed at the Public Health Laboratory—joined him in Cincinnati to become his wife. Their daughter, Susan, was born in that river city.

In 1916 a poliomyelitis epidemic of unprecedented magnitude swept the United States, and Frost, with others, was assigned to work on the problem. It was an appropriate task for him. In 1909, while working in the Hygienic Laboratory, he had transmitted polio to monkeys by direct inoculation, confirming the results of experiments carried out by Karl Landsteiner in Vienna, Austria, the preceding year. Frost had become interested in the disease at that time and had demonstrated that serum from convalescent polio patients protected experimentally infected monkeys. He concluded from this observation that the serum contained protective antibodies, the presence of which confirmed the diagnosis. He had conducted a number of studies of small polio outbreaks in Iowa, Ohio, and western New York State. Although polio had been recognized as infantile paralysis for a century, only with improved sanitation at the end of the nineteenth century had it become an epidemic disease affecting adults.[10] Frost's report of his studies in Iowa are remarkable for the thoroughness of the epidemiologic field investigation and, once again, for quantitative analysis of the large amount of data accumulated. His conclusions, while they fell short of what would later be learned of the epidemiology of poliomyelitis, were remarkably well founded and accurate; they reflected current contemporaneous thinking with origins in an epidemic in Sweden two decades earlier. "The infective agent," Frost noted with remarkable prescience, "is, during epidemics at least, quite widespread throughout the population affected, the incidence of the clinically recognizable disease being limited by the relatively rare susceptibility to the infection."[11]

In 1917 the United States entered World War I, and the mobilization of the country led to suspension of work at the Cincinnati laboratory. Frost, who had been promoted to the rank of Surgeon, drew an assignment to the Red Cross in Washington, where he organized its Bureau of Sanitary Service. However, his service there soon came to an end in November when he was found to have tuberculosis. The treatment of tuberculosis at that time centered on what was known as "the outdoor life" in locations where the climate was thought to be especially favorable. Among these spas was Asheville, North Carolina, where in 1875 Joseph Gleitsmann had established the first of many tuberculosis sanatoria soon to grace that mountain town. Frost went to Asheville, spending six months there before returning to light duty with the Public Health Service.

Whatever light duty meant to those who prescribed it for the recovering Frost, it did not mean a diminution of his energetic activities to him. Shortly after his return from Asheville, the great pandemic of influenza swept across the nation and the world. Probably beginning in American army training camps, it spread during the late summer and early fall of 1918 like a series of great tsunamis across the United States and especially among the civilian population of American cities. It traveled to Europe on troop ships. This epidemic took the lives of 675,000 Americans and killed more of the nation's soldiers than died in battle during the war. Frost was placed in charge of an epidemiologic study of the evolving plague. Among those assigned to work with Frost was a statistical economist, Edgar Sydenstricker, They became congenial colleagues, and the collaboration of these two pioneers was important in introducing statistical analysis into the growing science of epidemiology.

As they began their work, Frost, Sydenstricker, and their coworkers found it necessary to confront a lack of reliable information on the magnitude of the problem. It had been recognized in Europe some seventy years earlier that influenza epidemics were associated with an overall increase in mortality. However, this general observation gave little insight into the severity of the epidemic. Nevertheless, Frost later wrote, "Because of the incompleteness and lack of uniformity in reports of influenza morbidity, the only comprehensive statistical record of the recent pandemic must be based on records of mortality. While this deficiency of morbidity records is by no means peculiar to influenza, it is . . . a serious obstacle to broad epidemiological studies, which require for their basis accurate records of the occurrence of infection in various demographic units. Owing to the variable factor of case fatality, statistics of mortality alone do not afford an accurate measure of relative case incidence, so that analysis of mortality alone may fail to bring out important epidemiological features, or, still worse, may point to erroneous conclusions."[12]

Monthly mortality records for all forms of pneumonia and for influenza had been kept in Massachusetts beginning in 1887, and Frost noted that these records revealed winter month peaks coinciding with the influenza epidemic of 1890–1892. Similar peaks were found in more recent monthly mortality data for 1916–1918 from Cleveland, San Francisco, and New York City.[13] To this day, the United States Centers for Disease Control and Prevention provides week-by-week, state-by-state data on reported pneumonia deaths during the winter months in its weekly bulletin *Morbidity and Mortality Weekly Report* so that public health officers and practicing physicians can gauge the severity of the winter influenza season.

The solution to the problem posed by the lack of morbidity data was found in house-to-house surveys, and in December 1918, following the peak of the first wave of the national epidemic but before the second wave, such surveys were conducted in thousands of households in New London, Baltimore, Spartanburg, Louisville, Little Rock, San Antonio, and San Francisco. From these surveys data emerged that demonstrated that death rates were correlated closely with the incidence of pneumonia, with about thirty percent of influenza victims who developed pneumonia succumbing. Case fatality rates were highest in infants, young adults, and the elderly.[14] The organizational tasks for this study presented enormous challenges for Frost; so also did the handling of the large mass of data collected. The quantitative skills of Frost, Sydenstricker, and their colleagues were challenged but equal to the task. These studies may have represented Frost's earliest use of age cohorts to examine epidemiologic data, a tool that he later developed and used in his studies of tuberculosis.

The Johns Hopkins School of Hygiene and Public Health

Peace returned to the world in the fall of 1919. The leaders of all aspects of life in the United States returned to building the great institutions and industries that were expected to carry the nation forward. In Baltimore,

William Henry Welch returned to his dream of establishing a school of public health at the Johns Hopkins University. As its dean, he had catapulted the Johns Hopkins School of Medicine into a place of preeminence in medical education, recruiting an extraordinary medical faculty. He now wished to turn his attention to public health, an area of interest that had germinated in his mind while he was in New York, perhaps influenced by Hermann Biggs. As noted in Chapter 5, the world's first institute of hygiene world had been established in 1878 at the University of Munich by Max von Pettenkofer, an environmentalist who did not believe in the microbial origin of disease. When Robert Koch assumed his professorship of hygiene at the Institute of Hygiene of the University of Berlin, he introduced bacteriology and with it laboratory science to the field. Welch was also a scientist, and he had a science-based program in mind. In 1916 he had obtained a grant from the Rockefeller Foundation to establish an Institute of Hygiene and School of Public Health at Johns Hopkins. Now, with the war behind, he resigned his deanship to become director of the new School of Hygiene and Public Health.

Welch asked the man generally recognized as America's leading epidemiologist, Wade Hampton Frost, to join his new faculty. Welch also recruited the statistician Lowell Reed, and Frost and Reed quickly became friends and collaborators.[15] Working at first in scattered old buildings, the new faculty developed programs that became models for the teaching of public health worldwide. Frost was initially appointed as resident lecturer. He retained his Public Health Service commission, Welch having persuaded Surgeon General Hugh Cumming to assign Frost to the Johns Hopkins faculty. Later, in 1921, he became professor of epidemiology and then head of the Departments of Epidemiology and Public Health Administration. In 1929 he resigned his commission in the Public Health Service, and in 1930 he was elected dean of the School of Hygiene and Public Health by his faculty colleagues. With his reputation well established and continuing to grow, Frost accepted positions as scientific director of the International Health Division of the Rockefeller Foundation, as a member of the Advisory Council and Technical Board of the Milbank Memorial Fund, and as consultant in communicable disease control to the New York State Department of Health.

Much admired and revered by both faculty and students, Frost worked hard at his teaching role. He found lecturing difficult and discomforting. But he excelled in small-group teaching where his wit and his logical thinking were readily apparent to his students. He became known for his use of real-case problems as didactic tools. He stepped back from authorship, and allowed his students to publish much of the work which he had inspired. And his students went on to positions of importance in many venues.

Studies of Tuberculosis

Frost's interests gradually moved from the problems presented by the epidemiology of acute infectious diseases—typhoid, poliomyelitis, influenza—to the problems of chronic infectious diseases. Tuberculosis was perhaps the most important such disease of the time, and it had touched Frost's own life. Not surprisingly, Frost chose to attack this disease. The challenges presented were large and novel. Unlike most acute infectious diseases, tuberculosis is characterized by a variable and often long interval between infection and disease, and patients may be infectious for a substantial time period before their diagnosis is made. As noted below, Frost's longitudinal studies of tuberculosis pioneered in the use of two important epidemiologic techniques that dealt with this problem, the use of index cases as focal points for investigation and the study of age cohorts over long periods of time.

The Harriet Lane Clinic at Johns Hopkins Hospital, originally directed by Clemens von Pirquet (Chapter 7), began accepting tuberculous children from Baltimore in 1928. Frost recognized the potential of this clinic for providing epidemiologic information about tuberculosis, and he soon had his graduate students studying it. Theses by Miriam E. Brailey, R. E. Wheeler, C. H. Eller, and James Watt were concerned with the transmission of tuberculous infection and the morbidity and mortality of tuberculosis in these children.[16] In 1933 Frost himself worked to design forms and set norms for data collection in the clinic. The data thus collected formed the basis for a monograph published in 1958 by Miriam E. Brailey, the first of those graduate students.[17]

In 1930 Eugene L. Bishop, Tennessee's Commissioner of Health and a former graduate student of Frost, asked Frost to review data from

Tennessee. With that, his most important work on tuberculosis began, work that was to change forever not only the study of tuberculosis but the entire field of epidemiology. He and his graduate students, A. R. Foley, H. C. Stewart, J. A. Crabtree, and R. L. Gauld, first turned their attention to Gibson county, in western Tennessee, and then to Kingsport in the northeast corner of the state.[18]

The study in Kingsport was seminal, presenting unique challenges and resulting in new ways of thinking about the transmission of infectious diseases. "For the acute communicable diseases, such as diphtheria, scarlet fever, and measles," Frost noted, "measurement of the morbidity risk of familial contacts is a simple procedure, because the excess risk is concentrated within a few weeks following the invasion of the household."[19]

Not so, for tuberculosis. As he had done in his earlier studies of influenza, Frost turned to household surveys, and from these surveys emerged the concepts underlying the use of an index case as the starting point for investigation. Let us examine Frost's description of the problem and his methods:

> For tuberculosis the requirements are essentially the same [as for acute infectious diseases], but are more difficult to meet, chiefly because the disease is of slow evolution, and we cannot assume that the risk with which we are concerned is concentrated within the year or even the decade following establishment of the known exposure. It may, perhaps, be manifested by excessive morbidity or mortality in any subsequent period of life. Hence, observation of the exposed group must extend over a sufficient number of years to define the rates of morbidity and mortality prevailing in successive periods throughout the usual span of life. To keep a sufficiently large group of people under systematic, exact observation for such length of time is a difficult task which has, indeed, been undertaken in various places, but to the best of my knowledge has not been carried much beyond a decade. However, such simple facts as lie within the knowledge and memory of the average householder may be obtained by *retrospective* investigation, tracing familial histories backward into the past. The procedures followed in a preliminary attempt to apply data collected in this way and to check their reliability may be described best by referring to a concrete example.
>
> The available records which best serve the purpose of illustration are from a survey of the Negro population of Kingsport, Tenn., made during 1930 and 1931 by a special unit of the Tennessee State Department of Health.

The survey covered 132 families, constituting practically the entire Negro population of the city (The federal census Of 1930 gives the Negro population of Kingsport as 596. The persons living and present in the families surveyed numbered 556. Only three families are known to have been omitted (because of unwillingness to be examined), but it is probable that a few others may have been missed). For each family the investigation included a detailed familial history, extending as far back as practicable, and examination of every present member in a special clinic, where the routine procedure was: physical examination, roentgenogram of the chest, and tuberculin test. With very few exceptions, the full schedule of examinations was carried out for all persons, regardless of whether or not there was any reason to suspect tuberculosis.

In addition to numerous other items which do not come into the present discussion, each family schedule gave the following:

1. Date of establishment of the household, which may be defined more exactly as the date when the present head of the household came into that position. This is an important item, as it marks the date from which at least one informant may be expected to have first-hand knowledge of occurrences within the household.

2. A list, by name, of all persons present in the household when the schedule was made out, giving, for each person: familial relationship, date of entrance into household, age at time of investigation, record of any present or past illness diagnosed as certain or probable tuberculosis, record of clinic examination, and a detailed account as to time and circumstances of any known household contact with antecedent cases of pulmonary tuberculosis.

3. A list, by name, of all former members of the household, giving, for each: age at which entered the household, record of known or suspected tuberculosis while in the household, record of household contact with antecedent cases of phthisis; age at which withdrawn from the household, status when withdrawn—whether living or dead—and, if dead, date of death, with ascribed cause.

These records were made with great care, each family being revisited as often as necessary to check and complete the information; and as the families were thoroughly cooperative, it is believed that the facts within their knowledge were stated with fair accuracy. From the histories obtained, it is probable that the deaths ascribed to pulmonary tuberculosis actually were due to that cause; but it is by no means certain that these were all the deaths attributable to tuberculosis, and as to nonfatal cases of this disease the histories, both negative and positive, obviously are subject to considerable error. Also, the *early* history of *former* members, who were born outside of the households in which they were recorded, must often be unknown. However, in general, the facts are simple and, for the period since establishment of each household, presumably within the knowledge of the informant.[20]

What did Frost and his students do that made this study noteworthy? They covered a span of many years by relying on histories obtained by interview. They then traced the evolution of a microepidemic within a household starting with the first person known to have been diseased, the index case. Today, contact investigations, which health officers conduct following the recognition of a case of infectious tuberculosis, move forward and outward from that index case into the world of contacts of the patient. Frost, by working retrospectively, was able to extend this investigation over a time span of decades. Although he worked with the past, he produced a technique for looking forward.

Pioneering as the Kingsport study was, Frost's subsequent work in Williamson County, Tennessee, just south of Nashville, was even more important. This long-term study, undertaken with support of the Rockefeller Foundation, used the methods of the Gibson County and Kingsport studies with little modification. Managed by a team that included a number of Frost's former students, it began in 1931 and continued for twenty-four years, finally being reported in 1963 in a monograph published as a supplement to the *American Review of Respiratory Diseases*.[21] In a long memorandum dated November 13, 1931, Frost laid out the detailed plans for this study, clearly establishing his role as its architect.

Frost first turned his attention to the problems of defining morbidity and mortality rates over long periods of time. Drawing upon earlier studies of tuberculosis and making use of life table techniques used by insurance companies, he expanded upon the techniques he had introduced in the earlier Tennessee studies using modified life tables based on person-years. This required defining a starting point, and for this purpose he chose to use the index case, defined in the report of the study as "the person with known or suspected tuberculosis in a household who first came to the attention of the study and motivated the investigation of that household."[22] The importance of the index case in these longitudinal studies was discussed by the authors of the Williamson County monograph, Frost's former students, and it is worth reviewing here.

Concept of the index case: The onset of a disease like tuberculosis is difficult to pinpoint because symptoms may be vague or altogether absent for a considerable period of time following the development of a lesion. It is often impossible, therefore, to determine the "primary" case of tuberculosis in a household in which more than one case has occurred. The *first* person in a household who comes to the attention of medical or health authorities because of tuberculosis is a definite entity, around which the experience of other household members can be observed. Frost designated such an individual the "index case" because the discovery of this person led to the investigation of his household associates. The index case may or may not be the very first person with tuberculosis in a specific household, but it is the first known to the investigator. Often, investigation turns up other diseased persons in the same household, and it may be impossible to establish the chronology or sequence of disease occurrence, and therefore impossible to designate the "source" case. Without a primary case it is not proper to speak of "secondary cases" or "secondary attack rates" in the sense used by Chapin in his studies of acute communicable diseases. Furthermore, by using the index case to identify the people at risk, the whole universe of such people is included. This would not be true in those instances in which a "primary" case of tuberculosis had died and no current case of the disease was present.

The index case becomes the pivotal or focal person in a household, the frame of reference, so to speak. Everything of epidemiologic import that happens in the household is related to the date of investigation of the household (which coincides closely with the date of discovery of the index case). The individual members of the household are identified in terms of their relationship to the head of the household and to the index case. Antecedent experience is measured back in time from the date of investigation. Prevalence data are related to the date of investigation, and observational or incidence data start with that date.

The use of the index case served another, more subtle, purpose. The Kingsport Study showed up a hidden bias or "joker," as Frost liked to designate it. When a comparison was made of antecedent mortality in the study households and in the control population, the former group unexpectedly showed lower rates for the ages 26 to 49 years. The "joker" was discovered by Frost who showed that in the study households the antecedent history was given usually by a parent who had been present at the time of establishment of the household, and was obviously alive. In the control families, however, the "informant" was not necessarily a parent, but occasionally, a survivor of a family that was broken by the death of a parent. This situation tended to swell the antecedent mortality rate in the control families. By eliminating the adult informant from the study household population at risk the adjusted rates came into line with the expected rates.

By casting the index case in the role of the excluded "informant," bias in the calculation of antecedent mortality was eliminated. Frost also pointed out that the index case, since he already had tuberculosis, should also be eliminated from any calculation of future risk of morbidity and mortality; otherwise, bias in the direction of increasing the rates would be introduced. By the ingenious development of his concept of the index case, Frost was able to overcome several serious methodologic obstacles to the epidemiologic study of chronic disease.

The use of the index case in the present study was described in two early papers that reported on study findings.

Although both the index case and modified life-table concepts were developed and tested to some degree before the Williamson County Tuberculosis Study was initiated, their full utilization and exploitation were not achieved until Frost, as consultant to the study, built them into its program and personally observed their application to the longitudinal study of the chronic, infectious, communicable disease, tuberculosis.[23]

An elegant investigative approach, a novel and enduring way of viewing the spread of disease, a fundamental epidemiologic concept—these were the intellectual achievements of Frost that were clearly expressed in these studies of tuberculosis. They by themselves would have secured Frost his richly deserved place in the history of modern medicine. But more was to come from Frost's fertile mind.

In 1937 Frost published a paper remarkable for its time entitled "How Much Control of Tuberculosis?"[24] In this article he discussed much of his current thinking on the epidemiology and control of tuberculosis. He noted that tuberculosis was declining in incidence throughout the United States. He then stated, "for the eventual eradication of tuberculosis it is necessary only that the rate of transmission be held permanently below the level at which a given number of infection-spreading (i.e., open) cases succeed in establishing an equivalent number to carry on the succession. If, in successive periods of time, the number of infectious hosts is continuously reduced, the end result of this diminishing ratio, if continued long enough, must be extermination of the tubercle bacillus." In this statement he presaged the recent work of Roy M. Anderson and Robert M. May, who have made the general case that the ratio of average number of secondary infectious individuals resulting from primary infectious individuals to the average number of primary infectious individuals (designated R_0) must exceed 1.0 for the pathogen to survive.[25] This concept underlies much of modern mathematical modeling of infectious disease epidemiology and much of modern long-range planning for disease control.

As 1937 drew to a close, Frost was experiencing difficulty swallowing. Soon he was found to have a carcinoma of the esophagus. He was a heavy cigarette smoker, and it ironic that longitudinal cohort studies of the type introduced by Frost were later to be so important in demonstrating the association of this and other cancers with tobacco. Wade Hampton Frost died on May 1, 1938.

But the story of Wade Hampton Frost did not end with his death. In fact, his most notable paper, which has repeatedly been cited as a landmark in epidemiology, was published posthumously, assembled from his drafts by his colleagues and accompanied by his draft figures. Stating the problem that he wished to analyze, Frost wrote:

> As we pass along the age scale from infancy through childhood, to early adult life, and on to old age, the curve of mortality from tuberculosis shows a continuous movement either upward or downward. This is such a familiar fact that we are apt to take it for granted; to dismiss it as characteristic of the disease, and to pass on. But there is perhaps no single statistical record which is potentially of more significance. . . .
>
> But the record is peculiarly difficult to read with understanding, because it is immediately apparent that the most striking changes in mortality rate do not correspond to reasonably probable changes of like extent in rate of *exposure* to infection. For instance, nothing that we know of the habits of mankind and the distribution of the tubercle bacillus would lead us to suppose that between the first and the second five years of life there is, in general, a *diminution* in exposure to infection which corresponds to the decline in mortality rate. And there is little, if any, better reason to suppose that the extraordinary rise in mortality from age ten to age twenty, twenty-five, or thirty is paralleled by a corresponding increase in rate of exposure to specific infection.[26]

The decline in mortality in childhood and subsequent rise in young adulthood, referred to by Frost, had been elegantly demonstrated in Frost's studies in Tennessee. While he would now use data from Massachusetts, the roots of this paper were clearly implanted in Tennessee. Table 8.1 presents tuberculosis mortality data from Massachusetts from 1880 to 1930 in the form in which Frost assembled it. In his paper, Frost bracketed the data for the cohort born in the decade ending in 1880; I have used bold italics for this purpose in Table 8.1.

Tracking the 1880 cohort, one easily observes the peak mortalities in infancy and early adulthood. Frost went on to note that:

1. At every age mortality is lower in the later period.
2. In each period age selection is generally similar: mortality is high in infancy, declining in childhood, rising in adolescence to a higher level in adult life.
3. In the later period (1930) the highest rate of mortality comes at the age of fifty to sixty, whereas formerly it was at age twenty to forty. . . .

Commenting on these points, Frost observed that he wished:

. . . merely to call attention to the apparent change in age selection which has taken place gradually during the last thirty to sixty years, and to note that when looked at from a different point of view this change in age selection is found to be more apparent than real. . . .

Looking at the 1930 [data], the impression given is that nowadays an individual encounters his greatest risk of death from tuberculosis between the ages of fifty and sixty. But this is not really so; the people making up the 1930 age group fifty to sixty have, in earlier life, passed through *greater* mortality risks.[28]

Frost's paper included a number of figures illustrating his points. Figure 8.1 reproduces Figure 3A from his paper and illustrates the data for females for the cohorts of 1880 and 1930.

With great insight into not only the epidemiology but the pathogenesis of tuberculosis, Frost concluded:

1. Constancy of age selection (*relative* mortality at successive ages) in successive cohorts suggests rather constant physiological changes in resistance (with age) as the controlling factor.

Table 8.1
Death rates per 100,000 from tuberculosis, all forms, for Massachusetts,
1880 to 1930, by age and sex, as presented by Frost.[27]
Rates for the cohort of 1880 italicized.

Age	1880	1890	1900	1910	1920	1930
Males						
0– 4	*760*	578	309	209	108	41
5– 9	*43*	49	31	21	24	11
10–19	126	*115*	90	63	49	21
20–29	444	361	*288*	207	149	81
30–39	378	368	296	*253*	164	115
40–49	364	336	253	253	*175*	118
50–59	366	325	267	252	171	*127*
60–69	475	346	304	246	172	95
70+	672	396	343	163	127	95
Females						
0– 4	*658*	595	354	162	101	27
5– 9	*71*	82	49	45	24	13
10–19	265	*213*	145	92	78	37
20–29	537	393	*290*	207	167	92
30–39	422	372	260	*189*	135	73
40–49	307	307	211	153	*108*	53
50–59	334	234	173	130	83	*47*
60–69	434	295	172	118	83	56
70+	584	375	296	126	68	40

2.   If, as we may suppose, the frequency and extent of exposure to infection in early life have decreased progressively decade by decade, there is no indication that this has had the effect of exaggerating the risk of death in adult life due to lack of opportunity to acquire specific immunity in childhood.

3.   Present-day "peak" of mortality in *late* life does not represent postponement of maximum risk to a later period, but rather would seem to indicate that the present high rates in old age are the residuals of higher rates in earlier life.

With this paper in its original publication as a footnote (but unfortunately omitted from some of the subsequent republications) was a letter Frost had written to his old friend and colleague, Edgar Sydenstricker, in 1935. This letter substantially expands the analysis of the data presented. He wrote, in part:

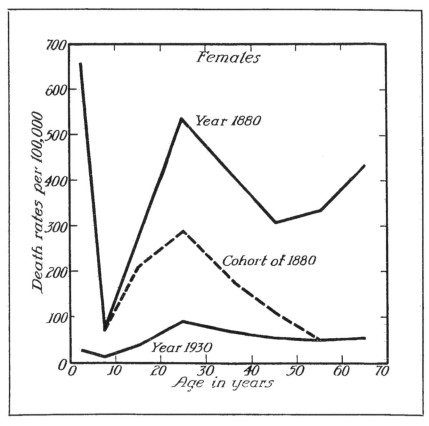

Figure 8.1. Massachusetts death rates for females from tuberculosis (all forms) by age, in the years 1880 and 1930 and for the cohort of 1880 as plotted by Frost. The broken line for the cohort of 1880 demonstrates clearly that the mortality seen in individuals in the sixth decade of life in 1930 was a legacy of the high infection rates in that cohort rather than a reflection of ongoing infections in 1930. Frost WH. The age selection of mortality from tuberculosis in successive decades. Amer J Hygiene 1939; 30:91–96. Figure reproduced with permission of the publisher.

For some years I have thought of the high mortality in later life as being related to *escape* from excessive mortality in earlier adult life. I have been thinking of the tuberculosis of today as a disease which has not the killing power to cause much mortality in the vigor of young adult life but becomes fatal in middle age or later when vital resistance has declined. It

has seemed to me that it was approaching the age-selection of pneumonia—fatal chiefly at the extremes of life, non-fatal in the more vigorous
ages. . . .

Viewed in this light [of the Massachusetts data] the relatively high
mortality rates now exhibited in the higher age groups seem to me to
have a significance quite different from what I had attributed to them.
They may be interpreted as the residuum of the much higher rates which
the now aged cohorts have experienced in earlier life. In general, the rule
seems to be that the higher the mortality of any cohort in early life, the
higher will it be in later years. Or, to have passed through a period of
high mortality risk confers not protection, but added hazard in late life.
. . .

All of this seems to me to have a bearing on the question which in
raised in the MS I sent you a few days ago—namely, how much if any
we may expect adult mortality to be increased as the result of dimin-
ished infection in the favorable years of childhood—from age 3 to 12. It
also seems to me to have a bearing on the moot question whether the
tuberculosis of adult life is almost wholly exogenous—due to recently
acquired infection—or to a considerable extent endogenous—the out-
cropping to clinical severity of infection which has remained latent or
smoldering through the childhood years when vital resistance seems to
be at its height . . .[29]

Clearly Frost understood tuberculosis in a fashion equalled by few of
his contemporaries and, indeed, by few modern students of the disease.

When Frost joined the Johns Hopkins faculty, the School of Hygiene and Public Health was housed in a number of older buildings in
Baltimore. One of them contained a stained glass window that included
Hotspur's words to the gentle Lady Kate: "Thou wilt not utter what
thou dost not know."[30]

Wade Hampton Frost was a seeker of the truth; he did not utter
what he did not know. His genius was that he found truth where others
looked but did not see. He introduced quantitative science to the previously empiric field of public hygiene, pioneering in its transformation
to the modern field of data-based, statistically analyzed epidemiology.

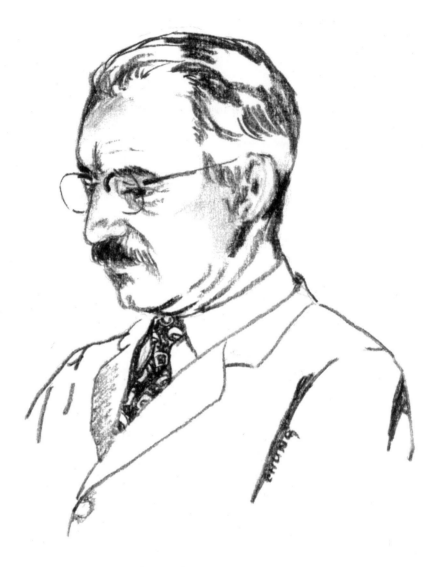

Selman Abraham Waksman

9

Selman Abraham Waksman
1888–1973
Pioneer of Antibiotics

The Renaissance and subsequent industrial revolution, which so dramatically altered the lives of Western Europeans and North Americans, scarcely crossed the Carpathian Mountains into the fertile land of the Ukrainian steppes. Indeed, much of Ukrainian life at the end of the nineteenth century was trapped in the middle ages. A polyglot region with an early history dominated by invasions of Huns from the East and Vikings and Poles from the West, the Ukraine with its rich top soil and favorable weather remained a region of small farms. While enjoying early prominence as Rus, one of the largest and most prosperous states of medieval Europe, with its capital in Kiev, its rural areas were largely untouched not only by the advancing civilization of Western Europe but also by the Czars who ruled from St. Petersburg and Moscow. Moreover, not only did the industrialization of western Europe fail to reach the Ukraine, but so also did the epidemic of tuberculosis that ravaged other parts of the continent during the eighteenth and nineteenth centuries bypass this eastern corner of Europe.

This rural region was the boyhood homeland of Selman A. Waksman, the eminent soil microbiologist who gave us the word "antibiotic." Waksman described the land of his birth as:

> Flat and surrounded by wide, forestless acres. In summer, the fields of wheat, rye, barley, and oats formed an endless sea. In winter, snow covered the ground, and the frosted rivers carried the eye to the boundless horizon, where the skies met the earth somewhere far away. Only the slow-flowing rivers and brooks, with occasional groves of oak and chestnut, broke this continuity of land and sky. The earth was black, giving rise to the very name for that type of soil, *tchernozem*, or black earth.

The soil was highly productive, yielding numerous crops, grown continuously for many years, without diminishing returns. . . . [1]

Selman Abraham Waksman was born on July 8, 1888. His mother named him Zolman (Solomon) after her father, a name which he later changed to Selman.[2] He was born in the town of Navaia-Priluka, a town which scarcely exists today, having been destroyed by the German armies that marched on Volgograd (Stalingrad) during World War II.

It was a bleak town, a mere dot in the boundless steppes. . . .

The town itself would hardly impress a visitor as worth a second glance. It had little if anything to offer to a city dweller. It was a small town. Very few of its inhabitants obtained from life more than a bare existence, and even that required hard, continuous struggle. In spite of the abundant crops and the well-fed herds of cattle and sheep, of swine and horses, and the hard-working people, life was materially poor, since the resources went to fill the coffers of the landlords, the Czar and his retinue, and the police. . . .

Just try to imagine the physical appearance of the town. Several parallel rows of whitewashed, straw-thatched adobe houses surrounded a large, open square, with a well at one corner. Here, on religious festivals or on market days, the peasants from the various villages would come to trade, to sell their agricultural produce, and to buy manufactured goods. They also came to meet friends and to make merry. Returning to their villages in their creaky, ungreased, horse- or ox-drawn wagons in summer, and in their smooth-running sleighs in winter, they left the square full of garbage and refuse. Then for several days, peasant women cleaned up the debris with their long-handled brooms made of reeds and rushes growing close to the local brook, and again the square was bare.[3]

A Jewish Boy

Askenazic Jews migrated from Germany and Prussia into the Ukraine during the fifteenth and sixteenth centuries, Waksman's ancestors among them. Waksman's life in Priluka was the life of a Jewish boy, Judaism influencing his family and community life in nearly every aspect. The Waksmans were tradespeople, not farmers, and deeply religious. They valued education and knowledge.

Little was known by Waksman of his paternal ancestry. His grandfather, Abraham, was a coppersmith, his father, Jacob, a weaver and upholsterer. Substantial landholdings had been inherited by his father, and he devoted more energy to managing these properties than to his trade. In fact, Waksman's parents lived separate lives, and his father was not often present in the family. Waksman remembered him best as "a storyteller" who imparted biblical knowledge to him but had only a minor role in his upbringing. In his autobiography Waksman devotes no more than a few scant paragraphs to him.

The family in which Selman Waksman spent his youth was, in his words, "a true matriarchate." The Waksmans were merchants in Priluka. Waksman's grandmother, Eva London, had been widowed at a young age, and she lived with the youngest of her six daughters, Fradia, Waksman's mother, who joined her in her mercantile efforts, importing a variety of goods for sale in the small town. Waksman had a sister, seven years his junior, who died at age two of diphtheria. Thus, the household in which Selman Waksman was raised was one headed by two women, and his kindred one that included five aunts.

Waksman's mother was determined to provide her young son with a rigorous classical and religious education. Public schools were not available, so Selman was enrolled in private ones. Finding these inadequate, she engaged private tutors to augment the boy's education. Not only did Selman learn the elements of reading and mathematics, of literature and history, but also of Jewish biblical history and the Hebrew language. He studied Yiddish literature and the Talmud, learning to recite long Biblical passages. Of his Jewish upbringing, Waksman wrote:

Who can ever describe the Day of Atonement in a poor synagogue in a small town in the Ukraine! The day when all the men and all the women spent their time in fasting and in praying for forgiveness of the sins they had committed during the year. That sacred music sung by the Cantor and his choir penetrated into every fiber of my small body and filled me with hopes for better days to come. Who can describe the happy festivals full of rejoicing, where one expressed the sentiments of his innermost self and identified himself with the Holy Writ, with the Holy Torah! Who can ever understand but one who has absorbed it through the pores of his whole body from his earliest childhood! . . .

I recall those days of prayer, with the men in the house of worship and the women of the neighborhood assembled in our home. They came to listen to my mother read and interpret to them the history of their people, a people who have given so much to the world, the Law, the principle of Justice, the very God himself[4]

The Russo-Japanese War of 1904–1905 was far removed from the Ukraine, but even in Priluka it had a major impact. Economic hardship was thrust upon the nation, and with it came unrest and agitation for a more representative form of government. Czarist agents descended upon the town, seeking evidence of sedition. The Waksman home was searched, and Waksman briefly jailed but promptly released when only religious tracts were found in the house. Although the young Waksman had socialist inclinations, he had never become involved in politics.

As Selman Waksman grew through the teenage years, he outstripped the schooling available in Priluka. Encouraged by his mother, he sought to enter a gymnasium in a nearby city. Admission was by examination, and most schools had few places for Jews. After failing to win entry in the nearby city of Zhitomir, he gained acceptance to the Latin Gymnasium in Odessa as an extern, or nonmatriculated, irregular student. He spent two years of study in Odessa and Vinnitsa and then passed the examinations and submitted a thesis to qualify for his diploma in 1910. This period in his life was marred by the death of his mother in the summer of 1909 of an intestinal obstruction, a surgical emergency for which no medical intervention was available in the small town.

University education in Russia seemed beyond Waksman's reach. The number of places available to Jews had become tightly constrained by quotas. Many young Jews went to Switzerland for higher education, and Waksman briefly considered this option. Following Fradia Waksman's death, a number of letters from members of the family—Selman Waksman's cousins—who now lived in America had arrived, and some of them encouraged him to think of immigration to that land. When Peisi Mitnik, his closest friend, agreed to join him, Waksman decided to emigrate and join his cousins in the land of promise. Peisi's sister, Deborah, called Bobili, would follow later, and Selman had already developed a romantic interest in this young woman, whom he would later marry.

Immigrant

With three men sharing a steerage bunk, Selman Waksman, Peisi Mitnik, and three others from Priluka embarked on a twelve-day voyage across the Atlantic from Bremen to Philadelphia where they were met by two of Waksman's cousins on November 2, 1910. Waksman went to Metuchen, New Jersey to live on the farm of cousins Mendel and Molki Kornblatt; Peisi Mitnik settled in New York. Waksman went to work on the Kornblatt farm, although farming activities were at a winter nadir, and devoted his spare time and energies to studying English.

Waksman, now twenty-two, was determined to obtain a university education, and his interests lay primarily in biology and life processes. He applied to and was accepted at the College of Physicians and Surgeons of Columbia University in New York, but he found the tuition costs daunting. He visited Rutgers University, only a few miles from the Kornblatt farm, and there he met Professor Jacob G. Lipman, also a Russian immigrant, who chaired the Department of Bacteriology. Lipman encouraged him to think of this field of study and of Rutgers, and when Rutgers offered him a scholarship, Waksman was quick to accept it.

University studies excited Waksman, especially the advanced science courses of his upper-class years, and his continued presence on and involvement with the daily activities of his cousin's farm fostered a growing interest in the vital processes of soil, manures, compost, and humus. He selected soil bacteriology for his major. In June 1913 Waksman accepted a caretaker job at a university farm. Housing was provided for him there, and in leaving the Kornblatt home he became more independent. He supplemented the income from this position by tutoring other immigrants in English. And he began traveling regularly to New York, where Bobili had joined her brother Peisi. Their romance flowered, but marriage would have to await the completion of Selman's studies.

Having carried more than the required course load, Waksman began his senior year with most of his bachelor's degree requirements completed. He devoted much of this last year of college to independent study and research with Professors Jacob Lipman and Byron Halstead, who became nurturing mentors for the bright young scientist. Waksman's senior research project was a study of the bacteriology of soil in relation to soil type and depth, and this survey first acquainted him with actinomycetes, the microorganisms to which Waksman would devote most of his extraordinarily productive scientific career. When Waksman was elected to Phi Beta Kappa late in his senior year, Halstead gave him the money to purchase a key. Later, Selman and Bobili Waksman would name their only son Byron Halstead Waksman.

Selman Waksman graduated from Rutgers in 1915. Lipman offered him an assistantship, and he stayed on as a graduate student to complete a masters degree the following June. Meanwhile, Lipman presented Waksman's soil survey data to the annual meeting of the Society of American Bacteriologists and published them in abstract in the *Journal of Bacteriology*. Together with his fellow graduate student and friend, Roland Curtis, Waksman published his data in February 1916, the first of his many papers.[5]

That spring, Selman Waksman became an American citizen. He also completed his masters degree work and applied to doctorate programs. He was accepted at several, and chose a program in chemistry at the University of California in Berkeley, attracted both by the studies in enzymology of T. B. Robertson, who would be his senior professor, and the size of the fellowship offered. The latter inducement would prove to be a hollow one, for upon arrival in California Waksman found even modest living costs to be substantially higher than could be met with funds from the fellowship.

Before departing for California, however, Selman Waksman journeyed to New York to marry Bobili on August 4, 1916. The next day the couple set off on the tedious cross-country train trip. They found California and Californians to be friendly and were soon settled in rented quarters. Professor Robertson was a disappointment, however, giving little attention or guidance to Waksman. In this situation, Waksman continued his studies of actinomycetes, focusing on their enzymes and those of fungi found in soil. To supplement his income, he took a position with Cutter Laboratories where he was placed in charge of a laboratory of ten to fifteen people preparing media and developing biological products and antisera. He completed his studies and was awarded the Ph.D. degree in 1918.

Professor of Soil Microbiology

Waksman and his wife returned to Rutgers upon completion of his graduate studies at Berkeley. He received an initial appointment as a lecturer at the Rutgers Agricultural College and microbiologist at the New Jersey Agricultural Experimental Station. He took up his post in the department of Jacob Lipman, his former mentor, and took charge of a section created for him by Lipman. He named his unit "soil microbiology," broadening the scope of Lipman's studies, which had been limited to bacteria, to a more comprehensive examination of soil microorganisms. His salary was small, smaller than that of his fellowship in California, and to supplement his income he took a position at Takamine Laboratories in Clifton, New Jersey. Jokichi Takamine, like Waksman an immigrant, successfully crystallized epinephrine in 1900, and he used the money derived from this discovery to create a commercial empire based on fertilizers and a variety of medicinal products.[6] He is perhaps remembered by nonscientists as the donor of the first three thousand cherry trees planted in Washington's tidal basin. At Takamine's New Jersey facility, Waksman was placed in charge of a laboratory conducting toxicity studies. He studied the toxicity of salvarsan, a mercurial used for the treatment of syphilis, an area of study he found challenging and one that may have had importance to his thinking as he later worked on antibiotics. In fact, this work was to become synergistic with studies of the compounds isolated in the Rutgers laboratory. In order to facilitate commuting to both of his positions, Waksman found it advantageous to move to New York City. One year following their return from California, Bobili gave birth to the Waksmans' only child, Byron Halstead Waksman.

Waksman's academic career at Rutgers developed steadily. In 1925 he was promoted to associate professor, in 1930, professor. In 1927 he published a fundamental text entitled *Principles of Soil Microbiology.*[7] In 1940, a Department of Microbiology was organized at Rutgers and Waksman was named to its chair. In 1949, he became director of Rutgers' newly created Institute of Microbiology.

Graduate students flocked to work with Waksman. Eleven students received advanced degrees under his tutelage during his first decade at

Rutgers; ultimately the number grew to seventy-six. He was a popular mentor. In a tribute written for Waksman's eightieth birthday, H. Boyd Woodruff, who was his graduate student and received the Ph.D. degree in 1942 for work that included the discovery of actinomycin, wrote of him:

> Each generation of students has its own memories of association with Dr. Waksman, a potpourri of effects on maturing men and women. Mine must be typical—watching Dr. Waksman at the laboratory bench each afternoon—conflicts at seminars over interpretations of data by biologists and physical chemists—tours of the Bowery taken to broaden students' appreciation of life—meeting the returning boat after his working vacations at a marine laboratory—unappreciated exhortations on learning the contributions of old masters—sharing in critiques at journal clubs—meeting the stream of dignitaries who visited the soil microbiology laboratory—gaining breadth from association with multilingual students from foreign lands—taking pride in his election as President of the Society of American Bacteriologists—enjoying departmental picnics at the Jersey shore—noticing the treasured companionship between the teacher and his Bobili. Our generation and those thereafter spoke fondly of the "Old Maestro." When this started, we do not know. Now that we have reached an age equivalent to his when he served as our teacher, we are amazed at our temerity. We recall that it was spoken in respect and love.
>
> Year after year has passed and associations grow richer. We realize that changes must come. No longer can students be guided, research be conducted. The imprint has been made. It will not be lost. It carries forward generation by generation, diluted to be sure, less recognizable as to origin. Like the waves of the sea it will ever grow broader, touching more and more, and never ending.[8]

Waksman's initial research upon his return to Rutgers represented a continuation of his earlier work with Lipman on the microbial ecology of soil, with emphasis on actinomycetes. It was largely descriptive, perhaps even pedestrian, not yet infused with the vision that pervaded his later studies of antibiotics. Waksman was busy preparing courses for which he was now responsible. Moreover, his work at Takamine Laboratories, his major source of income, was demanding.

Actinomycetes remained central to much of Waksman's science throughout his life, and it is worth digressing to consider Waksman's career in relation to these organisms. In the early eighteenth century, Carolus Linnaeus, a Swedish naturalist, developed a system for classifying all living forms. This system, which started with dividing life into kingdoms of plants and animals (additional kingdoms have been added recently) and progressed through various classes and orders to genera and individual species, has been amplified but has survived in its essential form to the present. It is used by all biologists, and individual life forms are named first by genus and then by species, according to the usage proposed by Linnaeus. Among the bacteria within the Linnaeus's kingdom of plants is the order Actinomycetales. While a few human and animal diseases such as actinomycosis and mycetoma have been associated with microorganisms of this order, most of its genera and species are nonpathogenic soil-living organisms. In many of their characteristics, they are organisms intermediate between bacteria and fungi. Waksman's first paper from his student days with Jacob Lipman had been devoted to these organisms, noting that they grew at a greater depth in the soil than other microorganisms.[9] On his return to Rutgers, Selman Waksman resumed his studies of actinomycetes. He returned home, not only to Rutgers but also to the soil and to those of its life forms that had first captured his attention.

Selman Waksman contributed importantly to the taxonomy of actinomycetes, and he and his students published many papers over several decades dealing with these microbes. Of seminal importance from his own student days in Lipman's laboratory, although it was given little attention at the time, was his and fellow student Roland Curtis's original isolation from California adobe soil of an organism they named *Actinomyces griseus*. They described its characteristics on five different culture media. On Cazpeck's agar medium it grew as:

> Colony round, 3 to 6 mm. in diameter, growing rapidly with the formation of numerous rings. Color of colony olive-buff. . . . Aerial mycelium appears at an early stage; it is a thick powdery mass of a water-green color. . . . The color of the aerial mycelium is somewhat lighter than that described by Krainsky. Odor present, but weak. Microscopically, the aerial mycelium is found to consist of long filaments, with very little

branching. These fragment readily into rod-shaped conidia, 1 to 1.5 x 0.8 . The conidia occur often in chains; they do not stain readily in the centre; so that they produce a beaded effect.[10]

A quarter of a century later, Waksman and Arthur Henrici described the genus *Streptomyces*, including in it *S. griseus*, reclassifying it from *Actinomyces* into this new genus.[11] This is the organism, rediscovered, that produced streptomycin.

Today it is easy to look back on Selman Waksman's career and his devotion to the actinomyces with a certain smugness, for we now can hardly doubt the importance of the organisms that gave rise to streptomycin and other antibiotics. However, when Waksman first threw himself into the study of actinomycetes and related soil microbes, the concept of antibiotics did not exist. Waksman was interested in the soil, and in his autobiographical writings he related this interest to his rural upbringing. But much more than that, Waksman was possessed of a scientific curiosity that transcended the practical world and medicinal remedies. Waksman was interested in soil microbiology, and he discovered streptomycin because he focused on actinomycetes—not the reverse. Waksman was in the truest sense a basic scientist, and his basic research produced unforeseen results of extraordinary benefit to humankind.

There appears to have been a degree of restlessness in Waksman's scientific mind during his early years at Rutgers. He attended scientific meetings and at them and at every other opportunity he sought out other microbiologists, seeking to learn all that he could from them. The modern reader must remember that only four decades had passed since Koch introduced solid culture media and oil immersion microscopy, the two fundamental techniques that first permitted the study of individual species of microorganisms; the community of scholars interested in these minute life forms was small.

In 1924, accompanied by Bobili, Selman Waksman returned to Europe. He attended an International Conference on Soil Science in Rome, finding much of it disappointing. "Met a lot of very curious people," he wrote, "who, under the guise of soil bacteriology or `microbiology,' a term that has not as yet come into popular use in Europe, manage to pull the wool over people's eyes and play politics. Some are bombastic.

They seem to know something of the earlier history of the subject, but not the latest contributions. They appear to be little interested in the subject. There are only a very small group, perhaps five or six, who are seriously interested in advancing our knowledge of soil microorganisms."[12] Yet, despite this disappointment, Waksman found his trip rewarding, and he took the opportunity to visit most of the major European bacteriologists and their laboratories.

Selman and Bobili Waksman took the opportunity presented by this trip to Europe to revisit their native Ukraine and Priluka. In the wake of the ravages of the Russian revolution, it was a heart-wrenching experience:

Finally we perceived the straw-thatched houses of Priluka! What a picture! Many were in ruins, most were shabby, and only few in fair condition. The people were in rags. There were large numbers of dirty children and elderly people; very few young and middle-aged men. Our entrance was like a triumphal procession. Everything alive poured out to meet us. I felt like falling to the ground and weeping, not sentimental tears, but the bitter tears of a son coming back to his motherland and finding her destroyed, her children reduced to the lowest state of degradation, their means of living gone. How can they be helped, and who is to help them?

I can no better express my feelings than by citing the entry in my diary, dated July 30, 1924, and written in Priluka itself:

"The greatest misery that one could ever imagine, the greatest catastrophe that the peoples in Russia have gone through; the greatest experiment in social and political relations of men can hardly express what we have seen during the last few days. Human life lost all vestige of value. A human being dressed in rags, living in a sometimes half-broken-down house, feeding on meat once a week. I have seen here, in the town where I was born and brought up, among the people whom I loved, human misery as it could only be imagined. The first impression was as if I were walking through a cemetery, with a few living ghosts wandering among the ruins. This misery overshadows by far in my thoughts the greatest experiment in human relations ever attempted, namely the communistic regime in Russia. It is rather difficult to decide with what to start; the head is full of impressions. Here I am sitting on a bench, a simple board on two projections, in front of the house, and looking upon the big open space, the center of Priluka. Near me is sitting Bobili Baron, my own Bobili's cousin. She, who formerly glorified in her education and

social position, is now a poor creature, dressed in rags, sitting or stand-
ing, quiet, not saying a word but merely looking on."[13]

Perhaps still not as scientifically focused as he would later become,
Waksman diverted his interest away from the actinomycetes to other
aspects of microbiology—to sulfur metabolism by soil microbes and to
the formation of compost, humus, and peat. In 1931 he organized a
division of Marine Bacteriology at the Woods Hole Oceanography Institute; he later became a trustee of the institute. With his family, he
spent many summers working at Woods Hole. During World War II
his laboratory at Woods Hole worked on the microbiology of the foul-
ing of ship bottoms.

Waksman was an early and vigorous protestor of the antisemitism
emerging in Germany during the 1930s, withdrawing from the editorial boards of German journals and refusing to participate in German
scientific congresses. He called the war, "the second world catastrophe."[14]
His son, Byron, served in the war in the European theater.

Antibiotics

It is above all for his work on antibiotics that Waksman is famous. The
earliest observations that certain substances could kill pathogenic microorganisms without harming the host were those of Paul Ehrlich.
Ehrlich was a dye chemist, and he observed that some dyes selectively
stained individual animal tissues without coloring others. Noting that
dyes also selectively stained microorganisms and being interested in trypanosomiasis, Ehrlich discovered that trypan red not only stained try-
panosomas but protected mice against the organism. Other animals,
however, were not protected. Ehrlich continued and eventually discovered salvarsan, an arsenical that not only provided effective treatment
for trypanosomiasis, but also cured syphilis. Ultimately, Ehrlich's work
provided the foundation for the discovery of sulfonamides in the 1930s,
the first chemical agents effective in treating many common infections.

That one microorganism could inhibit the growth of another was
probably first observed by Pasteur in 1877, and unsuccessful attempts
were made to isolate drugs useful in treating infections from microbes

as early as the late nineteenth century.[15] In 1929 Alexander Flemming had observed that an extract of the common mold *Penicillium notatum* had antibacterial properties. He named the active component penicillin, but he did not succeed in purifying useful quantities of it for further study. Howard Florey and Ernest Chain accomplished this task in 1939, revolutionizing the treatment of infectious diseases.

In 1923 Waksman coauthored a paper with one of his graduate students, Robert L. Starkey. They wrote in their introduction, "Certain soil organisms, including fungi, actinomycetes and bacteria produce substances toxic to the growth of others."[16] They referenced earlier observations by Grieg-Smith and by Nadson and Zolkiewicz. Perhaps this was the beginning of Waksman's realization that soil organisms might produce antibiotics. In a paper published in 1937, he and his graduate student Jackson W. Foster described the antagonism of actinomycetes and fungi to the growth of several bacterial species.[17] This antagonism was achieved using a filtrate of a strain designated *Actinomyces* 3065, with maximum antagonism produced by filtrates of seven- to eighteen-day-old cultures.

Waksman felt that the seminal event in the history of the development of modern antibiotics was not the discovery of penicillin, but rather the work of René Dubos. In an address given at the Mayo Clinic in 1944, Waksman reflected upon the origins of his interest in and thinking about antibiotics in the following terms:

> When I returned to Rutgers . . . certain ideas began to crystallize gradually in my mind. These laid the basis for the future development of the subject of antibiotics. Thus, in 1925 I found that a combination of two organisms leads to the formation, from proteins and amino acids, of products which are not formed by any one organism alone. In 1932, I received a grant from the National Research Council to study "the fate of acid-fast bacteria in the presence of free-living organisms of the soil, as providing the basis for a chemical study of a well-known group of bacteria which are of great economic importance in relation to one of the most common members of the natural population of the soil." Following a series of studies on the effect of one organism upon another in the decomposition of plant residues, I completed in 1936 a comprehensive investigation on the associative and antagonistic effects of microorganisms. These results emphasized the fact that actinomycetes are able

to exert a considerable influence upon the activities of fungi and bacteria in the soil.

Thus, toward the beginning of 1939, the various approaches to the subject of the interrelationships among microorganisms in the soil seemed to point to the advisability of my undertaking a detailed study of the effects of various microorganisms, notably the fungi and actinomycetes, upon disease-producing bacteria. . . .

Two events occurred that year which provided the necessary stimulus. *One was the work of a former student* [René Dubos, emphasis added, TMD] on the production by soil bacilli of substances (gramicidin, tyrocidine) which have a destructive effect upon disease-producing bacteria; I felt from my past experience that the fungi and actinomycetes would provide far more effective antibacterial agents than the bacteria. The second stimulus was provided by World War II, which was then looming on the horizon, and which pointed to a need for new agents for the control of various infections and epidemics that would no doubt arise.

After due consideration of the problem, I decided to direct my own efforts, and those of most of my graduate students and assistants, to the elucidation of the processes involved in the destruction by saprophytic soil microorganisms of bacteria causing human and animal diseases.

With the background of my work on soil microorganisms, it was only logical that I should turn to the soil in search of agents active against pathogenic bacteria. After various preliminary studies on the pyocyaneus organism as a producer of antibiotics, I gradually concentrated on the fungi and actinomycetes. The first antibiotic which we isolated in our laboratory in 1940, from a culture of an actinomyces, was designated as "actinomycin." The major importance of this discovery was the fact that it pointed to the possibility of utilizing actinomycetes as sources of antibiotics.

New methods for testing freshly isolated cultures of microorganisms for their antimicrobial potency were gradually developed or adapted from older procedures. The whole principle of screening was thus elucidated. With each subsequent step in the development of the antibiotics program in my laboratory, new progress was made in the understanding of the type of antibiotic that was wanted, and in methods for its production and isolation. Each new substance brought the final goal of obtaining proper chemotherapeutic agents nearer and nearer.[18]

In 1946 Waksman returned to Europe, and while in Sweden had an interchange that he later summarized as follows:

Another story is concerned with Prof. Lilienstrand, a brilliant pharma-cologist, who presided at Dr. Feldman's lecture. In discussing and sum-marizing this lecture, he commented as follows: "After a new discovery of gold, many people rush in order to collect the pebbles, and occasion-ally they find a gold nugget." The idea behind this statement was that after the discovery of penicillin, many people rushed to study antibiot-ics, and streptomycin was one such result. This was far from being the truth. But I could hardly respond to this discussion immediately. At the urgent request, however, of my friends in Stockholm, I wrote to Dr. Lilienstrand, assuring him that we had begun the study of antibiotics before the rediscovery of penicillin, that streptomycin had been isolated as a result of a rather difficult path that we followed and that had noth-ing to do with the discovery of penicillin. His simile was very brilliant, *but the gold rush should be traced to Dubos' isolation of gramicidin* [empha-sis added]; penicillin itself may have been one of the pebbles that he spoke about.[19]

Who was René Jules Dubos and what did he do that made Waksman place him at the origins of research on antibiotics? He was one of Waksman's earliest students. Having studied agronomy in Europe, he came to Rutgers as a graduate student in 1924. He soon became en-thralled with soil microbes, which he studied in Waksman's laboratory, and went on to obtain his Ph.D. with Waksman in 1927, working on cellulose decomposition by bacterial enzymes. Dubos then moved to the Rockefeller Institute and the laboratory of Oswald Avery, who hoped to find bacterial substances capable of attacking the polysaccharide cap-sule of pneumococci. There, he soon demonstrated that he could make highly virulent type III pneumococci susceptible to phagocytosis by stripping off its capsule with bacterial enzymes. In 1939 Dubos turned his attention to antibacterial substances produced by soil organisms, and he isolated the antibiotics tyrothricin and gramicidin. The tech-niques Dubos used were soon incorporated into studies in Waksman's laboratory, and they were of fundamental importance to Waksman's successful isolation of other antibiotics. Both of Dubos's drugs were used topically, but were too toxic for systemic use. Dubos went on later to study tuberculosis, contributing with his graduate student, Gardner Middlebrook, some of the standard culture media still in use for culti-vating *Mycobacterium tuberculosis*. And Dubos became a writer of note.

His *The White Plague*[20] became a classic, as did others of his works devoted to the social aspects of medicine.

As noted in Waksman's recollections cited above, work in Waksman's laboratory at the end of the 1930s and in the early 1940s became focused on the isolation of antibiotics from soil organisms. The discovery and rapid introduction into medicine of the miraculous penicillin was probably the major stimulus for this effort. René Dubos urged his former mentor to turn his attention to the products of actinomycetes, and the products of various of these organisms became the principal objects of study in Waksman's laboratory. Soon both actinomycin (in 1940) and streptothricin (in 1942) were purified. They proved to have broad antibacterial spectra, including gram-negative bacteria unaffected by penicillin, but they proved too toxic for clinical use. However, their isolation and the techniques developed in that work laid the foundation for further discoveries and for a new science devoted to antibiotics. In fact, the cell toxicity of actinomycin was later seized upon and the drug was used as a cancer-chemotherapeutic agent.[21]

Selman Waksman is generally credited with coining the term "antibiotic" in response to a query from T. B. Flynn, the editor of *Biological Abstracts*. Waksman's account of this coinage reads:

> Late in 1941 and early in 1942 it became apparent that we were dealing with a new field of science and that many new chemical compounds were about to appear, all of them possessing certain properties. This had begun with gramicidin in 1939, with the rediscovery of penicillin in 1940, and with our own isolation of actinomycin the same year. These were soon to be followed by a number of others. At the request of an editor of an abstract journal in 1941, I suggested the word "antibiotic" as an all-embracing term. In doing this, I made use of an old adjective, which was at one time used to designated the injurious effect of one organism upon another, as one preying upon another; in this respect the word had never come into general use. My suggestion was immediately accepted and received universal recognition. Before long, physicians spoke of "antibiotic therapy," pharmaceutical companies were organized as "antibiotic societies" [*sic*], and new journals dealing with "antibiotics" were started.[22]

Waksman, himself, appears to have first used the word "antibiotic" in a paper published with his graduate student and colleague H. Boyd Woodruff in 1942.[23] In fact, the origins of this word probably precede Waksman's use of the term. In 1941 and again in 1947, Waksman acknowledged the use of the terms "antibiose," antibiosis, and "antibiote", antibiotic (used as an adjective), in French papers as early as 1889.[24] In a prickly exchange of letters with Paul R. Burkholder published in 1952, Waksman appears to have forgotten his earlier citations as he claimed priority for the term.[25] In the 1953 letter, Waksman offered the definition of an antibiotic as, "a chemical substance, produced by microorganisms, which has the capacity to inhibit the growth and even to destroy bacteria and other microorganisms, in dilute solutions."[26]

The scale of Waksman's quest for antibiotics was enormous—an effort far greater than that usually mounted by research laboratories. In 1975, Waksman recounted:

> Together with my students and assistants, I have isolated and examined about 10,000 cultures of microbes from various natural substrates. Of these about 10 per cent, or 1,000, were found to possess antimicrobial properties. When these were grown in suitable media and the broths of these cultures tested, only about 10 per cent, or 100, were found able to produce antibiotics in the media. Each of these 100 antibiotics differed chemically from all the others. Since my facilities for chemical purification and identification were rather limited, we succeeded in isolating and describing only 10 per cent, or 10 of them.[27]

Streptomycin:
The "Magic Bullet" against Tubercle Bacilli

In May 1942 Waksman's son. Byron, then a medical student at the University of Pennsylvania, wrote to his father:

> In reading the reprints you sent me, I was struck again with the urge to do some work in the direction of finding an effective *in vivo* antagonist to the tubercle bacillus. I was particularly impressed with the relative simplicity of the method you have used in isolating fungi-producing antibiotic substances, and I wondered if exactly the same method could not be used with equal ease to isolate a number of strains of fungi or actinomycetes which would act against *M. tuberculosis*.[28]

Waksman was not quite ready for this challenge, however, but about a year later he turned to the task. In fact, as early as 1932, he had observed that tubercle bacilli were able to multiply in sterile soil but not in soil containing fungi, a clue which he failed to pursue at that time.[29] In June 1943 Waksman attended a small meeting in Philadelphia at which work on enzymes capable of attacking tubercle bacilli was presented. He thought this approach to have little promise for the treatment of tuberculosis, but was stimulated by the report to seek antibiotics effective against the cause of the white plague.

The details of how that search proceeded and ultimately succeeded with the discovery of streptomycin are obscured by inconsistencies among the writings of the principals and others who have recounted the story. At the root of this pernicious weed of distortion is the bitter enmity between Waksman and his graduate student, Albert Schatz, which culminated in a court suit. Waksman's several accounts all tend to stress the antecedents prior to the advent of Schatz and the role of many persons in his laboratory and elsewhere in developing the ideas upon which the work was based and the methods used in isolating streptomycin. Waksman's accounts also tend to be less than candid in discussing his financial gain from the discovery. Schatz's story, as told from interviews by Frank Ryan, focus on the enormous amount of effort that he put into the work.[30] They down-play the beginning graduate-student status and subordinate intellectual role of Schatz. Ryan, of course, did not have the opportunity to interview Waksman. Schatz felt that he was cheated of economic returns due to him and of recognition in the Nobel Prize award. In fact, Waksman may have had little or no opportunity to influence the Swedish Nobel Prize committee in its deliberations concerning the awardees of the prize.[31]

Albert Schatz had been an undergraduate at Rutgers, a brilliant student elected to Phi Beta Kappa in his junior year, a student majoring in microbiology and well known to Waksman. Schatz returned to Rutgers and Waksman's laboratory on June 30, 1943, as a Ph.D. candidate. Waksman put him to work searching for antibiotics. Less than two months later, he isolated streptomycin from an actinomycete designated *Streptomyces griseus*.[32] As noted previously, this organism had been originally isolated and described as *Actinomyces griseus* by Waksman and Curtis while they were students, and it had been recently reclassified as *S. griseus* by Waksman and Henrici. The strain used by Schatz was cultured from the throat of a chicken and originally studied by Doris Jones, another student in Waksman's laboratory; another isolate of *S. griseus* from soil proved to produce even greater concentrations of the antibiotic. Schatz used a technique of cross-streaking on an agar plate strains of actino-mycetes being screened with test organisms the growth of which might be inhibited by products secreted by the actinomycete. This technique was well established in the laboratory before Schatz's arrival. Once it was recognized that Schatz's isolate of *S. griseus* produced an antibiotic that had a broad spectrum of activity and was relatively nontoxic to animals, many other students and colleagues at Rutgers joined in the study of streptomycin. Notable among them was Elizabeth Bugie, who joined Schatz and Waksman as coauthor on the first published descrip-tion of streptomycin; F. R. Beaudette, the animal pathologist who had made the original cultures of the chicken's throat; and Doris Jones.

The first publication describing streptomycin appeared early in 1944; Schatz was first author, Elizabeth Bugie second, and Waksman third.[33] Although the new antibiotic was found to exhibit bacteriostatic activity against *M. tuberculosis*, little note was made of this activity in the paper. Later that year, the antibacterial activity against tubercle bacilli and other bacteria of streptomycin was compared with that of six other antibiot-ics in terms of dilution units per gram of dry, ash-free material.[34] Once again, Schatz was the first author and Waksman the second. Table 9.1 presents the results obtained with streptomycin.

The data in Table 9.1 appear to reveal some disparities. In fact, there may have been differences in the susceptibilities of individual cultures of bacteria used in the two sets of experiments, and the dilution units may have given different results in broth and plate cultures. What is remarkable, however, despite differences in strains and techniques, is that streptomycin was as effective against tubercle bacilli as it was against many common bacteria. No other agent with such potency had been previously described.

William H. Feldman was an experimental pathologist and bacteri-ologist at the Mayo Clinic. He had tested sulfonamides and other anti-infectives against tubercle bacilli, only to find them inactive. But his interest continued, and he was aware that Waksman was isolating anti-biotics from soil microorganisms. He contacted the Rutgers scientist,

Table 9.1

Antibiotic activity against *M. tuberculosis* and other bacteria as reported in early papers from Waksman's laboratory. Results are presented as dilution units, with broth cultures used in the earlier experiments and plate cultures used in the later ones. Data from Waksman, Bugie, and Schatz and from Waksman and Schatz.[35] I have assigned the strain designations H37Ra and H37Rv to the strains of *M. tuberculosis* used in the two studies summarized in this table on the basis of Ryan's description.[36]

Organism	Initial report	Second report
Pseudomonas aeruginosa	9,500	300
Escherichia coli	38,000	2,000
Bacillus mycoides	63,000	7,500
Bacillus subtilis	380,000	25,000
Mycobacterium phlei	320,000	10,000
Mycobacterium tuberculosis (H37Ra)	250,000	
Mycobacterium tuberculosis (H37Rv)		3,000
Mycobacterium avium	3,800	
Staphylococcus aureus		1,500
Shigella gallinarium		2,000
Salmonella pullorum		3,000
Serratia marcescens		2,500

and his letter resulted in an invitation to visit Waksman's laboratory.[37] In November 1943, at the time when streptomycin was being studied by Schatz, Bugie, and Waksman, Feldman made his visit to Waksman's laboratory in New Jersey. Following this visit, in January 1944, Feldman was excited to read the first account of streptomycin. Even before he could ask for some of the new drug, Waksman wrote to him asking him if he would be able to test it in his animals, and in April 1944 Waksman gave him ten grams of the newly isolated, but still crude agent. Together with his biologist-physician colleague Corwin Hinshaw, he tested streptomycin in four tuberculous guinea pigs with a series of injections beginning on April 27. Streptomycin proved to be both nontoxic and remarkably effective therapeutically. Then, dramatically, Hinshaw and Feldman administered the new antibiotic to a young woman dying of tuberculosis at the Mineral Springs Sanatorium in Cannon Falls, Minnesota. She recovered her health, almost miraculously. More patients followed, also with good responses, and chemotherapy for the disease that had become known as the Captain of Death was born.[38]

Streptomycin was not the only early drug effective in the treatment of tuberculosis. Other and better drugs would emerge later. But the antibiotic isolated by Schatz, Bugie, and Waksman stands historically in the van of the armamentarium of effective agents. Jorgen Lehman, in Sweden, discovered para-amino salicylic acid in 1943, almost simultaneously with the discovery of streptomycin. Gerhard Domagk, who was awarded the Nobel Prize in 1939 for the discovery of Prontosil, the first of the sulfonamides, but prevented from accepting it by the Nazi government of Germany until 1947, discovered tibione (thioacetazone) in 1944; it is still used as a low-cost companion drug for treating tuberculosis in some developing countries. Both of these drugs were the products of thoughtful chemistry, of a search for analogues or derivatives of sulfonamides that might affect mycobacteria. Both were bacteriostatic agents that were less efficacious than streptomycin and other subsequently discovered agents, and both would assume secondary roles in the treatment of tuberculosis. Neither was the major advance that streptomycin was; neither was the product of innovative conceptualization that streptomycin was; and neither received the worldwide immediate acclaim that streptomycin did. Nor did Lehman and Domagk share in the adulation that Waksman received.

Fame and the Nobel Prize

Waksman was a hero. As noted previously, the Waksmans went to Europe in 1946. This trip was a triumphal tour, and Waksman was received with honors at major universities and institutes throughout the continent. They made a similar trip in 1950. On many occasions they met patients, often children, who had been cured by streptomycin. Selman Waksman became the recipient of twenty-two honorary doctoral degrees and sixty-seven prizes, awards, and medals. These included the Lasker Award in 1948, the Nobel Prize in Medicine or Physiology in 1952, and the Trudeau Medal in 1961.

In March 1950 Albert Schatz filed suit against Selman Waksman and the Rutgers Research and Endowment Foundation. He sought public acknowledgement of his role in the discovery of streptomycin, an accounting of royalties received and their distribution, and half of the money thus earned. Waksman portrayed himself as dumbfounded by this event, but, in fact, Schatz, who had left the laboratory in 1946, had corresponded with Waksman and his attorneys over the assignment of patent rights and had not received straightforward answers to his questions.[39] Ultimately the suit was settled with the payment of $125,000 and three percent of the royalties to Schatz.

In the ceremonies presenting Waksman for the Nobel Prize, Professor A. Wallgren of the Karolinska Institute introduced Waksman and his work, noting the contributions of several coworkers including Albert Schatz, and then said:

> By the discovery of streptomycin Dr. Waksman and his collaborators have made a very important contribution to the history of medicine. Even if streptomycin is not the perfect anti-tuberculous remedy, its introduction nevertheless signifies a gigantic step forward. Above all, its isolation has suggested procedures for future investigations that may guarantee fundamental results. One may hope that this approach will lead in the near future to the eagerly expected goal, viz. a remedy that will make possible the eradication of tuberculous disease.[40]

In accepting the prize, Waksman reviewed the history of the discovery of streptomycin, the chemical structure and toxicity of streptomycin, the antibacterial spectrum of the drug, and its role in treatment of tuberculosis. "Medical science and clinical practice have been revolutionized," he said. "One may look forward to further discoveries of agents that will combat diseases not now subject to therapy."[41] He noted that many other antibiotics had already been discovered and entered medical use. In closing, Selman Waksman thanked some eighteen individuals working in his laboratory, including Albert Schatz, for their contributions. The trip to Sweden to accept the Nobel Prize provided the opportunity to continue around the world, and the Waksmans were received with honors in Japan and elsewhere in Asia.

That Flicker of Light That Has Left Its Trace

What does one do after receiving the Nobel Prize and making a triumphal world tour? For Selman Waksman, the answer was obvious. He returned to his laboratory. Of course, the laboratory had changed. Using money from streptomycin royalties, Rutgers had built the Lipman Institute of Research and named Waksman as its director when it opened in 1954. He wrote prolifically, some fifteen books appearing in the post-Nobel years, including his autobiography, *My Life with the Microbes*, and his reflective, largely autobiographical exposition, *The Conquest of Tuberculosis*.

Life after the Nobel Prize for Selman Waksman meant the search for additional antibiotics. Ultimately, some twenty-two of these wonder drugs would come from his laboratory. The only other one to come into clinical medical use was neomycin. An aminoglycoside, it was effective against *M. tuberculosis* and had a limited application in the treatment of tuberculosis. It had the renal toxicity characteristic of all aminoglycosides, and was not absorbed orally. It was used for preoperative bowel sterilization and remains one of the active ingredients of the commonly employed topical preparation, "Neosporin."

Waksman continued to spend his summers studying marine biology at Woods Hole. There, on August 16, 1973, at the age of eighty-five, he died suddenly of a cerebral hemorrhage.

Selman Waksman concluded his autobiography, *My Life with the Microbes*, with an introspective poem entitled "A Speck of Dust." The last stanza reads:

> I am that speck
> From the beginning of time
> To the end of time,
> That tiny speck in eons of time,
> That flicker of light
> That has left its trace
> Upon the course of life,
> The significance of which
> In this universe of time
> Is still to be unraveled.[42]

PART 3

Epilogue

"Will you walk a little faster?" said a whiting
    to a snail,
"There's a porpoise close behind us, and he's
    treading on my tail.
See how eagerly the lobsters and the turtles all
    advance!
They are waiting on the shingle—will you
    come and join the dance?
Will you, won't you, will you, won't you,
    will you join the dance?
Will you, won't you, will you, won't you,
    won't you join the dance?"

Lewis Carroll
"The Lobster Quadrille"

10

Reflections

Were a boy to find a penny one day, he might consider himself lucky. Were he to find two pennies on the next day, he might consider himself doubly lucky. Were he to double his luck every day, he would find more than five dollars on the tenth day, more than five thousand dollars on the twentieth day, and more than five million dollars on the thirtieth day. Such is the awesome way that exponential growth escalates. In this instance, the doubling time is a short one day. When I was a college student and enrolled in a biology class, one of the laboratory exercises required me to start a colony of fruit flies in a small bottle containing nutrient agar, carefully counting the flies each day. Just as did the trove of pennies found by the boy, the number of fruit flies grew exponentially. Part of the exercise was to calculate the doubling time, which I no longer recall. Then the population growth tapered off. The fruit flies had reached the maximum number that the contained ecosystem of the bottle could sustain—the limit. In fact, the number of pennies found by the boy would soon have to taper off as it reached the capacity of the government mints to produce new coins.

Science has been growing exponentially, just as did the pennies and fruit flies, with each century and each decade seeing more new knowledge acquired than did earlier periods. One might suppose that ultimately we will know everything about everything and growth of knowledge will stop, but that possibility is beyond our imagining. What we can imagine is that the next few decades will eclipse the enormous growth of medical knowledge that the lives of our pioneers—Laennec to Waksman—encompassed.

What will be the biomedical fields in which this new knowledge will appear? Molecular genetics? Biochemistry? New vaccines? More sophisticated statistically based interpretation of clinical and clinical trial data? Pharmacology? All of these and more.

What will impose limits on the growth of medical knowledge? Certainly, money will be one limiting factor. As research becomes more complex and more dependent upon frontier technology, it also becomes more expensive. The world's largest funder of biomedical research is the United Sates Public Health Service National Institutes of Health. In Frost's time it conducted research only in its own laboratories. While its intramural research programs continue and are now large, the agency began making extramural grants to research scientists in the years following World War II. That support has continued, but the amount of money in real dollars made available by the American tax payers has not kept pace with the growing costs of research. There have been years when fewer than one-fifth of scientifically merit-worthy projects have been funded. In more prosperous years, about one-third of proposed investigations passing peer review have received support.

Are the costs of scientific research justified? They are now large. Could the money be better spent on social programs, on military programs, on building roads? Who can place a value on the discovery of insulin in 1922 by Frederick G. Banting and his student Charles H. Best?[1] Prior to the introduction of vaccination programs, the United States witnessed nearly fifty thousand cases of smallpox and more than fifteen thousand cases of paralytic poliomyelitis annually.[2] Both of these scourges are now gone—smallpox from the entire world and polio from the Americas with the world soon to follow. During the first fifteen years following its introduction, isoniazid treatment of tuberculosis saved Americans nearly four billion dollars, more than six times the amount spent during the same time by the National Institutes of Health for research and training in all infectious diseases.[3] Christopher Murray, who has used elegant modeling techniques to study the epidemiology of disease and its impact on the world's economy, wrote in 1991, "In terms of costs per death averted and per year of life saved, chemotherapy for smear-positive tuberculosis is the cheapest health intervention available in developing countries."[4] Insulin, vaccines, and drugs are some of the products of biomedical research. Yes, the costs are justified, large as they may sometimes seem.

A major limitation on the advancement of biomedical science is and increasingly will be the training of new investigators. Just as for biomedical research itself, the National Institutes of Health has been the principal funder for the training of the scientists who will do the research. Just as money for research has often been tight, so have funds to support training often been scarce.

Of more fundamental importance than money, however, is the very problem of the expansion of knowledge. When I opened my research laboratory, I had under my belt two years of postdoctoral research training, and I was knowledgeable in and current with the techniques of the broad field of immunology. When I retired and closed my laboratory more than thirty years later, my knowledge and skill had become limited to a small segment of the field—partly because my own interests were then more sharply focused, but also because it was no longer possible for even the most diligent scientist to remain current in all aspects of immunology. With the passage of further time and the further expansion of knowledge, emerging new scientists will have to be sharply focused, both in training and in research effort. However, this narrow focus imposes another limitation. When I retired after more than three decades in the laboratory, I was beginning to feel the onset of obsolescence, even though I had made great effort to stay current in my field, even though my laboratory was busy and well funded, even though the problems I was then attacking and the approaches and techniques I was then using could not have been imagined when I began, and even though I was still producing and publishing important new data. That lurking cloud of obsolescence will descend earlier upon those whose basic research training is more highly focused.

Finally, let us stop for a moment and consider the limitation imposed by the communication of knowledge. New knowledge is of no use unless it is communicated. Laennec gave lectures and wrote books. Waksman did the same, but he also presented his work at scientific meetings and published his data in scientific journals; all of those means of communication are the norms of today. It is a paradox, however, that Waksman was able to have the published description of streptomycin in print within a few months of the wonder drug's discovery, but today, with all of our more modern means of communication, it typically takes a year or more for such exposition in print. Selection of a paper for presentation at a meeting now usually requires a submission of an abstract nine months or more in advance. Part of the problem is that the flood of new knowledge is so great that journal editors and program committees find it important to insist on peer review before publication at a time when the peers—other scientists—are so busy keeping their own projects on track that they find it hard to provide rapid review.

Some believe that posting of research data on the Internet is the solution, and in the physical sciences that practice has become common. However, such an approach by-passes peer review, which, for all the time it requires, provides much of value to scientist-authors and their readers. And reliance on the Internet and computer-dependent modes of knowledge transmission eliminates an important archival aspect of the dissemination of scientific knowledge. It should be obvious to readers of this book that I studied papers written more than a century ago in ancient volumes now preserved in medical libraries as I prepared my text. To those who think that information posted or stored using modern computer equipment will be accessible to the next generation of scientists, I issue the challenge of trying to play the music on some of my classic "thirty-threes" or trying to use any computer older than about ten years. What does one do today with information on a five-and-one-quarter-inch floppy diskette? How does one play an eight-track audio-tape?

The problem—problems, in fact—created by the rapid expansion of knowledge are confounded further by the broadening scope of knowledge and the broader purview required of a successful scientific investigator. As scientists must, perforce, become more sharply focused in their individual research efforts, they must also be familiar with an extraordinarily broad reach of science related to their work and potentially offering new insights and new opportunities for them. This type of mind expansion is best accomplished by personal interactions not dissimilar to those of Koch and Cohn or Feldman and Waksman. Email will certainly facilitate such dialogue, but it is unlikely to replace scientific colloquia and visits to the laboratories of colleagues. It is person-to-person communication that builds a community of scholars, and it is in such communities that new ideas flourish.

Who will lead us through the rapidly accelerating and increasingly complex scientific maze that I have projected? Who will be the pioneers of coming generations? Indeed, who are the pioneers of today? (I quite deliberately chose not to include living persons in my book.) Can we learn something from the lives of those who have preceded us? I believe so. Indeed, I would not have written this book were I not firmly convinced that we can. It should be valuable, then, to look at what the six pioneers profiled here had in common.

The six men of this volume were all clearly unrestrainable geniuses. While they all ascended from scientifically and sometimes personally modest antecedents, they rose to stand out above their contemporaries and peers. And they were recognized in their time by prestigious appointments and awards, including the Nobel Prize for Koch and Waksman. Their thinking was innovative and imaginative. They knew how to frame a hypothesis or a question so that it could be tested or answered, frequently using new techniques that they devised. They often transcended their own training; only Waksman among them had any formal training specific to the tasks later set. They were all critical thinkers. Are there such geniuses abroad in the biomedical scientific community today? Will there be tomorrow? Of course, there are and will be.

Each of the pioneers I have profiled devoted major effort to the training of young scientists who would follow behind and then move forward, in turn, to lead. The training and nurturing of those aspiring to research careers is one of the most productive efforts undertaken by scientists. It is also one of their greatest obligations. Indeed, it is an obligation for all who benefit from science—for all of us.

Notes

Chapter 1: Pages 3-16

1. Hippocrates. Book I. Of the epidemics. In Major RH. Classic descriptions of disease. With biographical sketches of the authors. Third edition. Springfield, IL: Charles C. Thomas, Publisher, 1945:52.

2. Fracastorius H. The theory of infection. Chapter II. Concerning the fundamental differences of contagions. In Major RH. Op. cit:8.

3. Sand G. George Sand and Chopin. A glimpse of Bohemia (a letter written to M. Francois Rollinat dated March 8, 1839; translated by Lewis Buddy). Canton, PA: The Kirgate Press, 1902.

4. Daniel TM. Captain of death. The story of tuberculosis. Rochester, NY: University of Rochester Press, 1998:71–2.

5. Budd W. The nature and the mode of propagation of phthisis. Lancet 1867; 2:451–2.

6. Koch R. The Nobel lecture on how the fight against tuberculosis now stands. Lancet 1906; 1:1449–51.

7. Ibid.

8. Riley RL, O'Grady F. Airborne infection. Transmission and control. New York, NY: The Macmillan Company, 1961. This slim volume provides an elegant summary of the work of Wells, Riley, and others who contributed to the understanding of airborne infections.

9. Chapman JS, Dyerly MD. Intrafamilial transmission of tuberculosis. Am Rev Respir Dis 1964; 90:48–60. See also Daniel TM. Op. cit:92–6 for further discussion of this subject.

10. Hyge TV. Epidemic of tuberculosis in a state school, with an observation period of about 3 years. Acta Tuberc Scand 1947; 21:1–57.

11. Riley RL, Mills CC, Nyka W, Weinstock N, et al. Aerial dissemination of pulmonary tuberculosis. A two-year study of contagion in a tuberculosis ward. Am J Hyg 1959; 70:185–96.

12. Van Leeuwenhoek A. Microscopic observations about animals in

the scurf of the teeth. Phil Trans Royal Soc London 1684; 14:568–74. Reprinted in Brock TD. Milestones in microbiology. Englewood Cliffs, NJ: Prentice-Hall, Inc, 1961:9–11.

13. Doetsch RN. Benjamin Marten and his "New Theory of Consumptions." Microbiol Rev 1978; 42:521–8.

14. Myers JA. Captain of all these men of death. Tuberculosis historical highlights. St. Louis, MO: Warren H. Green, Inc, 1977:29–31.

15. Metchnikoff E. The founders of modern medicine. Pasteur. Koch. Lister. New York, NY: Walden Publications, 1939:120–1.

16. Myers JA, Steele JH. Bovine tuberculosis control in man and animals. St. Louis, MO; Warren H. Green, Inc., 1969. Rosenkrantz BG. The trouble with bovine tuberculosis. Bull Hist Med 1985; 59:155–75.

17. Brock TD. Robert Koch. A life in medicine and bacteriology. Washington, DC: American Society for Microbiology Press, 1999:129.

18. Daniel TM. Op. cit:131–55.

19. Ibid:121–4.

20. Shoemaker SA. Mummies, mycobacteria, and molecular biology—The old and the new. Am Rev Respir Dis 1986; 134:642–3. Bloom BR. Tuberculosis control in the coming decades. An ordinary mortal's guide to the molecular biology of mycobacteria. Bull Internat Union against Tuberc Lung Dis 1989; 64:50–8.

Chapter 2: Pages 17-24

1. Chretien J. La tuberculose. Parcours imagé. Tome I. Propos. Auchel, France: Hautes de France, 1995:55.

2. Clifford JL. Young Sam Johnson. New York, NY: McGraw-Hill Book company, 1955. Wiltshire J. Samuel Johnson in the medical world. Cambridge, England: Cambridge University Press, 1991.

3. Schiff B. A line as clear and tensile as a lightning flash. Smithsonian 1994; 24:64–73.

4. Sargent S. Galen Clark. Yosemite guardian. Yosemite, CA: Flying Spur Press, 1981.

5. Sargent (ibid) describes Muir as consumptive. Wolfe's definitive biography of Muir describes him as healthy at the time of his joint

activities with Clark at Yosemite but chronically ill in later life at his ranch in Martinez. The nature of this illness is not specified by Wolfe, but it was marked by weight loss and cough, suggesting a diagnosis of tuberculosis. Wolfe LM. Son of the wilderness. The life of John Muir. Madison, WI: The University of Wisconsin Press, 1973. Originally published by Alfred A. Knopf, Inc., 1945.

6. I have written on the pathogenesis of tuberculosis in several publications intended for different readers. For physicians, medical students, and other advanced health professionals, more detailed information can be found in Daniel TM. Tuberculosis. In Isselbacher KJ, Wilson JD, Martin JB, Fauci AS, Kasper DL (editors). Harrison's principles of internal medicine, 13th edition. New York, NY: McGraw-Hill, 1994:710–8. Other standard medical texts also treat tuberculosis in generally satisfactory fashion. For those with less medical background, a more general treatment for nonprofessional readers can be found in Daniel TM. Captain of death. The story of tuberculosis. Rochester, NY: University of Rochester Press, 1998.

7. Vidal S, Trembley M, Govoni C, Cauthier S, et al. The Ity/Lsh/Bcg locus: Natural resistance to infection with intracellular parasites is abrogated by disruption of the Nrampl gene. J Exp Med 1995; 182:655–66. Lavebratt C, Apt AS, Nikonenko BV, Schalling M, Schurr E. Severity of tuberculosis in mice is linked to distal chromosome 3 and proximal chromosome 9. J Infect Dis 1999; 180:150–5.

8. Daniel TM, 1998. Op. cit:133–42.

9. Grzybowski S, Enarson DA. The fate of cases of pulmonary tuberculosis under various treatment programmes. Bull Internat Union against Tuberc 1978; 53:70–5.

10. Alling DW, Bosworth EB. The after-history of pulmonary tuberculosis. VI. The first fifteen years following diagnosis. Am Rev Respir Dis 1960; 81:839–49.

Chapter 3: Pages 25-33

1. Dickens C. Nicholas Nickleby. London: Penguin Books, 1986:731–2. Originally published in 1839.

2. Dubos R, Dubos J. The white plague. Tuberculosis, man, and society. Boston, MA: Little, Brown and Company, 1952:58.

3. Richman M. The man who made John Harvard. Harvard Magazine 1977; 80:46–51.

4. Moss A, Marvel E. The legend of the Latin quarter. Henry Mürger and the birth of Bohemia. New York, NY: Beechhurst Press, 1946.

5. Strouse J. The unknown J. P. Morgan. The New Yorker, March 29, 1999:66–79.

6. Hayman J. Mycobacterium ulcerans: An infection from Jurassic time? Lancet 1984; 2:1015–6.

7. Kapur V, Whittam TS, Musser JM. Is *Mycobacterium tuberculosis* 15,000 years old? J Infect Dis 1994; 170:1348–9.

8. Hare R. The antiquity of diseases caused by bacteria and viruses. A review of the problem from a bacteriologist's point of view. In Brothwell D, Sandison AT (editors). Diseases in antiquity. A survey of the diseases, injuries and surgery of early populations: 115–31. Bates JH, Stead WW. The history of tuberculosis as a global epidemic. Med Clinics N Amer 1993; 77:1205–17. Haas F, Haas SS. The origins of *Mycobacterium tuberculosis* and the notion of its contagiousness. In Rom WN, Garay SM (editors). Tuberculosis. Boston, MA: Little Brown and Company, 1996:3–19. Stead WW. Tuberculosis in Africa. Int J Tuberc Lung Dis 1998; 2:791–2.

9. Brown L. The story of clinical pulmonary tuberculosis. Baltimore, MD: Williams & Wilkins Company, 1941:3.

10. Morse D. Tuberculosis. In Brothwell D, Sandison AT (editors). Diseases in antiquity. A survey of the diseases, injuries and surgery of early populations. Springfield, IL: Charles C. Thomas, 1967:249–71.

11. Ibid:4.

12. Badger TL. Looking backward. Medical Dimensions, June 1976:8–11.

13. Deuteronomy 28:22; Leviticus 26:16; Psalms 106:15; Isaiah 10:16. The Holy Bible. Revised standard version. New York: Thomas Nelson and Sons, 1953. The Holy Bible. King James Version. New York: Collins' Clear-Type Press, 1937. In both of these English versions of the Bible, the translators of the passages in Deuteronomy and Leviticus used the word "consumption," from the Latin *consumptio* (a wasting and especially as used by both Ovid and Cicero a wasting disease) to translate the Hebrew word *schachepheth*, a wasting disease. This word persists in modern Hebrew as *schachefet*, the word for tuberculosis. At

the time of the English translations of the Bible, "consumption" was generally understood to mean tuberculosis. The Hebrew word used in Psalm 106 and Isaiah is razon, leanness or wasting from disease. In the Revised Standard Version, this word was translated in the two passages as a "wasting disease" and "wasting sickness," respectively. In the King James Version, the translators used "leanness" in both instances. For a more complete discussion of Biblical references to tuberculosis, see Daniel VS, Daniel TM. Old Testament Biblical References to Tuberculosis. Clin Infect Dis 1999; 29:1557–8.

14. Morse D. Op. cit; Morse D, Brothwell DR, Ucko PJ. Tuberculosis in ancient Egypt. Am Rev Respir Dis 1964; 90:524–41; Cave AJE. The evidence for the incidence of tuberculosis in ancient Egypt. Brit J Tuberc 1939; 33:142–52.

15. Cave AJE. Op. cit.

16. Zimmerman MR. Pulmonary and osseous tuberculosis in an Egyptian mummy. Bull NY Acad Sc 1979; 55:604–8.

17. Daniel TM. The early history of tuberculosis in central East Africa: insights from the clinical records of the first twenty years of Mengo Hospital and review of the relevant literature. Int J Tuberc Lung Dis 1998; 2:784–90.

18. Grayson DK. Confirming antiquity in the Americas. Science 1998; 282:1425–6. The dating of the Monte Verde site has been challenged by some. Pringle H. New questions about ancient American site. Science 1999; 286:657–8. However, whether the Monte Verde site dating is correct or is off by a few thousand years and whether it precedes other Clovis sites by one thousand years or not are not material to the point that the Americas were widely peopled prior to the opening of the Bering Strait and prior to domestication of animals.

19. Allison MJ, Mendoza D, Pezzia A. Documentation of a case of tuberculosis in pre-Columbian America. Am Rev Respir Dis 1973; 107:985–91. Arriaza BT, Salo W, Aufderheide AC, Holcomb TA. Pre-Columbian tuberculosis in northern Chile: molecular and skeletal evidence. Am J Physical Anthropol 1995; 98:37–45. Salo W, Aufderheide AC, Buikstra J, Holcomb TA. Identification of *Mycobacterium tuberculosis* DNA in a pre-Columbian Peruvian mummy. Proc Natl Acad Sci USA 1994; 91:2091–4. Daniel TM. The origins and precolonial epide-

miology of tuberculosis in the Americas: can we figure them out? Int J
Tuberc Lung Dis 2000; 4:395–400.

20. Allison MJ, Mendoza D, Pezzia A. Op. cit.

21. Salo W, Aufderheide AC, Buikstra J, Holcomb TA. Op. cit.

22. Morse D. Prehistoric tuberculosis in America. Am Rev Respir
Dis 1961; 83:489–504. Buikstra JE, Cook DC. Pre-Columbian tuberculosis in west-central Illinois: prehistoric disease in biocultural perspective. In Buikstra JE (editor). Evanston, IL: Northwestern University Archeological Program, 1981:115–39. Perzigian AJ, Widmer L.
Evidence for tuberculosis in a prehistoric population. JAMA 1979;
241:2643–6. Widmer L, Perzigian AJ. The ecology and etiology of skeletal lesions in late prehistoric populations from eastern North America.
In Buikstra JE (editor). Evanston, IL: Northwestern University Archeological Program, 1981:99–113. Pfeiffer S. Paleopathology in an
Iroquoian ossuary, with special reference to tuberculosis. Am J Physical
Anthropol 1984; 65:181–9.

23. Morse D, 1967. Op. cit. Ponce Sanginés C. Tenupa y Ekaku. La Paz,
Bolivia: Los Amigos del Libro, 1969. Daniel TM. An immunochemist's
view of the epidemiology of tuberculosis. In Buikstra JE (editor). *Prehistoric Tuberculosis in the Americas.* Evanston, IL: Northwestern University Archeologic Program, 1981:35–48.

24. Bates JH, Stead WW. Op. cit. Stead WW, Eisenach KD, Cave
MD, Beggs ML, Templeton GL, Thoen CO, Bates JH. When did *Mycobacterium tuberculosis* infection first occur in the new world? An important question with public health implications. Am J Respir Crit Care
Med 1995; 151:1267–8. Haas F, Haas SS. Op. cit.

25. Hippocrates. Book I. Of the epidemics. In Major RH. Classic
descriptions of disease. With biographical sketches of the authors. Third
edition. Springfield, IL: Charles C Thomas, 1945:52.

26. Daniel TM. Captain of death. The story of tuberculosis. Rochester, NY: University of Rochester Press, 1997:17.

27. Ulrich-Bochsler S, Schäublin E, Zeltner ThB, Glowatzki G.
Invalidisierende Wirbelsäulenverkrümmung an einem Skelettfund aus dem
Frühmittelalter (7./8. bis anfan 9. jh). Ein Fall einer wahrscheinlichen
Spondylitis tuberculosa. Schweiz Med Wschr 1982; 112:1318–23.

28. Myers JA. Captain of all these men of death. Tuberculosis his-

torical highlights. St. Louis, MO: Warren H. Green, 1977. Long ER. The decline of tuberculosis with special reference to its generalized form. Bull Hist Med 1940; 8:819–43.

29. Grigg ERN. The arcana of tuberculosis. With a brief epidemiologic history of the disease in the U.S.A. Amer Rev Tuberc Pulm Dis 1958; 78:151–72, 426–53, 583–603.

30. Holmberg SD. The rise of tuberculosis in America before 1820. Am Rev Respir Dis 1990; 142:1228–32. Waksman SA. The conquest of tuberculosis. Berkeley, CA: University of California Press, 1964:20.

31. Wilson LG. The historical decline of tuberculosis in Europe and America: Its causes and significance. J Hist Med Allied Sc 1990; 45:366–96. Davies RPO, Tocque K, Bellis MA, Rimmington T, Davies PD. Historical declines in tuberculosis in England and Wales: improving social conditions or natural selection? Int J Tuberc Lung Dis 1999; 3:1051–4.

32. Waksman SA. Op. cit:181.

33. Grigg ERN. Op. cit. Bates JH, Stead WW. Op. cit. Davies RPO, Tocque K, Bellis MA, Rimmington T, Davies PD. Op. cit.

34. McKeown T. A historical appraisal of the medical task. In McLachlan G, McKeown T (editors). Medical history and medical care. A symposium of perspectives. London: Oxford University Press, 1971:29–55. For additional discussion by the author of McKeown's thesis, see Daniel TM, 1997. Op. cit:37–8.

35. Reichman LB. The U-shaped curve of concern. Am Rev Respir Dis 1991; 144:741–2.

36. Dolin PJ, Ravigliione MC, Kochi A. Global tuberculosis incidence and mortality during 1990–2000. Bull World Hlth Org 1994; 72:213–20.

37. Ibid.

38. Pablos-Méndez A, Raviglione MC, Laszlo A, Binkin N, et al. Global surveillance for antituberculosis-drug resistance, 1994–1997. New Engl J Med 1998; 338:1641–9.

39. Neville K, Bromberg A, Bromberg R, Bonk S, Hanna BA, Rom WN. The third epidemic—multidrug-resistant tuberculosis. Chest 1994; 105:45–8.

40. Kipling R. The ladies. A Kipling pageant. New York, NY: Halcyon House, 1942:916–8.

Chapter 4: Pages 36-61

1. There are many available biographical accounts of Laennec's life. I have relied principally on the following: Webb GB. René Théophile Hyacinthe Laennec. New York, NY: Paul B. Hoeber, Inc, 1928. Kervran R. Laennec. His life and times. New York, NY: Pergamon Press, 1960. Hale-White W. Translation of selected passages from De l'auscultation médiate (first edition) by R. Théophile H. Laennec with a biography. New York: William Wood, 1923. Duffin J. To see with a better eye. A life of R.T.H. Laennec. Princeton, NJ: Princeton University Press, 1998. More concise accounts are given by many writers, including: Sakula A. In search of Laennec. J Royal Coll Phys London 1981; 15:55–7. Sakula A. RTH Laennec 1781–1826. His life and work: A bicentenary appreciation. Thorax 1981; 36:81–90. O'Shea JG. Rene Laennec: His brilliant life and tragic early death. Scot Med J 1989; 34:474–7. Keers RY. Laennec: his medical history. Thorax 1981; 36:91–4. Nuland SB. Doctors. The biography of medicine. New York, NY: Vintage Books, 1988:200–37. Webb's book is of particular interest because it draws upon and quotes extensively from the biography by Rouxeau, which was published in two volumes in 1912 and 1920 and for which an English translation is not available. Kervran's work is well researched and scholarly; it contains many details not found in other sources I have consulted. Hale-White's biography is also scholarly and adds further insights. Duffin's biography is elegantly researched and includes material from Laennec's papers and lectures that has not been available to other biographers. Duffin emphasizes the medical and historical context in which Laennec lived and worked.

2. Webb GB. Op cit. Kervran R. Op. cit. Long ER. A history of pathology. New York, NY: Dover Publications, Inc., 1965:76–81. Rapoport J. Laennec and the discovery of auscultation. Israel J Med Sc 1986; 22:597–601.

3. For an account of Guillaume Laennec's efforts to secure support for Laennec from his father, see Duffin J, 1998. Op. cit:22–3.

4. Duffin J, 1998. Op. cit:37. These remarks by Laennec must be taken in their proper context. They are from a letter rejecting his father's request for an appeal to Corvisart on the father's behalf. They may also be clouded by professional rivalries that developed between the two physicians.

5. Duffin JM. Sick doctors: Bayle and Laennec on their own phthisis. J Hist Med Allied Sc 1988; 43:165–82.

6. Duffin J, 1998. Op. cit:35–6.

7. Kervran R. Op. cit.

8. Jarcho S. The manuscript consultation reports of Francesco Torti. Bull hist med 1998; 72:73–4.

9. For a scholarly discussion of the subject, see Duffin J, 1998. Op. cit:124–8.

10. Sakula A, 1981a. Op. cit. Laennec RTH. A treatise on the disease of the chest, translated by Forbes J. Facsimile of the London 1821 edition. New York, NY: Hafner Publishing Company, 1962:284–5. As used by Laennec, the term mediate auscultation meant auscultation with an intermediate instrument—the stethoscope—as opposed to direct or immediate auscultation during which the examiner's ear was applied directly to the skin of the patient.

11. Laennec RTH. Forbes translation. Op. cit:437.

12. Duffin J, 1998. Op. cit:288–91.

13. Among Clark's famous tuberculous patients were Frédéric Chopin and John Keats. See Daniel TM. Captain of death: The story of tuberculosis. Rochester, NY: University of Rochester Press, 1997.

14. Laennec RTH. Forbes translation. Op. cit.

15. Ibid:ix.

16. Laennec RTH. Hale-White translation. Op. cit. 17. Ibid:34–5.

18. Ibid:42–3.

19. Laennec RTH. Forbes translation. Op. cit:1–11.

20. Pectoriloquy was recognized as a sign of consolidation by Victor Collin in 1823. See Duffin J, 1998. Op. cit:137.

21. Laennec RTH. Hale-White translation. Op. cit:32–3.

22. Laennec RTH. Forbes translation. Op. cit:307.

23. Long ER. Op. cit:82.

24. Long ER. Op. cit:114–26.

25. Duffin J. Vitalism and organicism in the philosophy of R.-T.-H. Laennec. Bull Hist Med 1988; 62:525–45.

26. Duffin J, 1998. Op. cit:174.

27. Sakula A, 1981b. Op. cit.

28. Weisz G. The posthumous Laennec: creating a modern medical hero, 1826–1870. Bull Hist Med 1987; 61:541–62.

29. Webb GB. Op. cit:ix–xi.

30. Brown L. The story of clinical pulmonary tuberculosis. Baltimore: Williams and Wilkins Company, 1941:22.

31. Duffin doubts this pregnancy. See Duffin J, 1998. Op. cit:256–8.

32. I have chosen to recount Laennec's medical history in the terms favored by most authorities, and thus I have ascribed most of his illness to tuberculosis. This position seems reasonable to me. There are dissenting views, however. Laennec almost certainly had asthma, and much of his symptomatology in Paris probably reflected this disease; some have considered asthma the cause of all or most of Laennec's medical problems. Others have suggested that most of his symptoms could be attributed to chronic sinusitis. Some writers have suggested he died of infective endocarditis. For discussions of possible causes of Laennec's illness other than tuberculosis, see: Keers RY. Op. cit. Also see O'Shea JG. Op. cit.

33. Kervran R. Op. cit:24–5.

34. Duffin JM, 1988. Op. cit:178.

35. O'Shea JG. Op cit. Laennec RTH, cited by Duffin JM, 1988. Op cit:179. Daniel TM. Percutaneous inoculation tuberculosis (letter). Clin Infect Dis 1998; 26:1486.

36. Laennec RTH. Lecture at the Collège de France. Quoted by Thayer WS. Osler and other papers. Baltimore: The Johns Hopkins Press, 1931:260.

Chapter 5: Pages 62-97

1. Porter JR. Louis Pasteur sesquicentennial (1822–1972). Science 1972; 178:1249–54.

2. Doetsch RN. Benjamin Marten and his "New Theory of Consumptions." Microbiol Rev 1978; 45:521–8.

3. Major RH. Classic descriptions of disease with biographical sketches of the authors, third edition. Springfield, IL: Charles C. Thomas. 1945:66–8.

4. Metchnikoff E. The founders of modern medicine: Pasteur, Koch, Lister. By Elie Metchnikoff. Including Etiology of wound infections by Robert Koch, The antiseptic system by Sir Joseph Lister, and Preven-

tion of Rabies by Louis Pasteur. Translation of Trois foundateurs de la médecine moderne. New York, NY: Walden Publications, 1939:9–11.

   5. There have been many biographies of Koch. Among them, I have found especially useful the scholarly and very readable Brock TD. Robert Koch. A life in medicine and bacteriology. Madison, WI: Science Tech Publishers, 1988. Dr. Brock is a distinguished microbiologist who brings to his writing not only facility with words but unique insights into Koch's work. I recommend this biography to all readers interested in Koch. Other major sources consulted include Metchnikoff E. Op. cit; Robinson V. Pathfinders in Medicine. New York, NY: Medical Life Press, 1929 and Robinson V. Robert Koch (1843–1910). Medical Life 1932; 39:129–87; Webb GB. Robert Koch (1843–1910). Ann Med Hist 1932; 4:509–523; Brown L. Robert Koch. Bull NY Acad Med 1932; 8: 558–84; Grange JM, Bishop PJ. Über tuberkulose. A tribute to Robert Koch's discovery of the tubercle bacillus, 1882. Tubercle 1982; 63:3–17; and Carter KC. Essays of Robert Koch, New York, NY: Greenwood Press, 1987. (Material from Carter reproduced with permission of Greenwood Publishing Group, Inc.) Alex Sakula has published three major papers on Koch: Sakula A. Robert Koch (1843–1910): Founder of the science of bacteriology and discoverer of the tubercle bacillus. A study of his life and work. Br J Dis Chest 1979; 73:389–94; Sakula A. Robert Koch: Centenary of the discovery of the tubercle bacillus, 1882. Thorax 1982; 37:246–51; and Sakula A. Robert Koch: The story of his discoveries in tuberculosis. Irish J Med Sc 1985; 154 (Suppl 1):3–9. Less scholarly biographies containing much personal material, much of which must be considered apocryphal, are the well known De Kruif P. Microbe hunters. New York, NY: Harcourt Brace & Company, 1926:101–39 and Knight DC. Robert Koch. Father of bacteriology. New York: Franklin Watts, Inc., 1961.

   6. Webb GB. Op. cit.

   7. Brock TD. Op. cit:24.

   8. Koch R. Die aetiologie der milzbrand-krankheit, begründet auf die entwicklungsgeschichte des Bacillus anthracis. Beiträge zur Biologie der Pflanzen 1876; 2:277–310. Translated in Carter KC. Op. cit:1–17. Carter's work provides English translations of Koch's major papers and makes these important papers available to Anglophones who do not read German.

9. Robinson V. 1929. Op. cit:718.

10. Ibid:719.

11. Cited by Smith T. Koch's views on the stability of species among bacteria. Ann Med Hist 1932; 4:524–30.

12. Brock TD. Op. cit:73.

13. Koch R. Untersuchungen über die aetiologie de wundinfection-skrankheiten. Lepizig: Georg Thieme, 1878. Translated in Carter KC. Op. cit:19–56.

14. Bulloch W. The history of bacteriology. London: Oxford University Press, 1936:227–30.

15. Bunyan J. The life and death of Mr. Badman. New York, NY: R.H. Russell, 1900.

16. Daniel TM. Captain of death: The story of tuberculosis. Rochester, NY: University of Rochester Press, 1997.

17. Krause AK. Tuberculosis and public health. Am Rev Tuberc 1928; 18:271–322; McKeown T. Medicine and world population. J Chron Dis 1965; 18:1067–77; Wilson LG. The historical decline of tuberculosis in Europe and America: Its causes and significance. J Hist Med and Allied Sciences 1990; 45:366–96.

18. Koch R. Die aetiologie der tuberculose. Berliner klinische wochenschrift 1882; 19:221–30. Translated in Carter KC. Op. cit:83–96. This landmark paper has been translated by many authors. I have used Carter's translation throughout.

19. Ibid. An excellent, scholarly account of Koch's work and the techniques he employed is given by Brock TD. Op. cit:117–26.

20. Ibid.

21. Webb GB. Op. cit:516.

22. An excellent discussion of Koch's postulates, their origins, and the importance of Koch's articulation is provided by Carter KC. Koch's postulates in relation to the work of Jacob Henle and Edwin Klebs. Med Hist 1985; 29:353–74. See also Doetsch RN. Henle and Koch's postulates. ASM News 1982; 12:555–6.

23. Brock TC. Op. cit:180.

24. Landis HRM. The reception of Koch's discovery in the United States. Ann Med Hist 1932; 4:531–7; Sakula A. 1982. Op. cit; Sakula A. 1985. Op. cit; Gröschel DHM. The etiology of tuberculosis: A tribute to Robert Koch on the occasion of the centenary of his discovery of

the tubercle bacillus. ASM News 1982; 48:248–50; Maulitz RC. Robert Koch and American medicine. Ann Int Med 1982; 97:761–6.

25. Koch R. Die aetiologie der tuberkulose. Mittleilungen aus dem Kaiserliche Gesundheitsamte 1884; 2:1–88. Excerpts translated in Carter KC. Op. cit:129–50.

26. Sattler EE. A history of tuberculosis from the time of Sylvius to the present day. Being in part a translation, with notes and additions, from the German of Dr. Arnold Spina. Containing also an account of the researches and discoveries of Dr. Robert Koch and other recent investigators. Cincinnati, OH: Robert Clarke & Co, 1883:150–1.

27. Daniel TM. Op. cit:178–94.

28. Trudeau EL. An autobiography. Philadelphia, PA: Lea and Febiger, 1916:175–6.

29. Trudeau EL. Environment in its relation to the progress of bacterial invasion in tuberculosis. Am J Med Sc 1887; 84:118–23.

30. Brock TD. Op. cit:140–68.

31. Koch R. An address on cholera and its bacillus. Brit Med J 1884; 2:403–7, 453–9.

32. Modern American readers should recall that in the Europe of Koch's day and, indeed, in much of the world today, academic departments had only one professor, and a professorial chair was a seat at the pinnacle of a pyramid of individuals with lesser-ranked academic appointments.

33. Brock TD. Op. cit:183.

34. Metchnikoff E. Op. cit:119–22; Heifets L. Metchnikoff's recollections of Robert Koch. Tubercle 1982; 63:139–41.

35. Koch R. Ueber bakteriologische forschung. Verhandlungen des X internationalen medizinischen kongresses. Translated in Carter KC. Op. cit:179–86.

36. Ibid.

37. Koch R. A further communication on a remedy for tuberculosis. Brit Med J 1890; 2:1193–5.

38. Dr. Koch's remedy for tuberculosis (editorial). Brit Med J 1890; 2:1200–1.

39. Anonymous. Character sketch. Dr. Robert Koch. Review of reviews 1890; 2:547–51.

40. Lister J. Koch's treatment of tuberculosis. Lancet 1890; 2:1257–9.

41. Doyle AC. Dr. Koch and his cure. Review of reviews 1890; 2:552–6.

42. Official report on the results of Koch's treatment in Prussia. Brit Med J 1891; 1:598–600.

43. Bothamley GH, Grange JM. The Koch phenomenon and delayed hypersensitivity: 1891–1991. Tubercle 1991; 72:7–11.

44. Koch and his critics, Spurious Koch's fluid (editorials). JAMA 1891; 16:59,61. Reprinted in JAMA 1991; 265:48.

45. Burke DS. Of postulates and peccadilloes: Robert Koch and vaccine (tuberculin) therapy for tuberculosis. Vaccine 1993; 11:795–804; Shapiro E. Robert Koch and his tuberculin fallacy. Pharos 1983; 46:19–22.

46. Metchnikoff E. Op. cit:118.

47. Sakula A. 1979. Op. cit.

48. James T. Professor Robert Koch in South Africa. S Afr Med J 1970; 44:621–4; Blumberg L. Robert Koch and the rinderpest. S Afr Med J 1989; 76:438–40; Brock TD. Op. cit:241–5.

49. Koch R. The Nobel lecture on how the fight against tuberculosis now stands. Lancet 1906; 1:1449–51.

50. Packer RA. Veterinarians challenge Dr. Robert Koch regarding bovine tuberculosis and public health. J Am vet Med Assoc 1990; 196:574–5.

51. Koch R. 1906. Op. cit.

52. Maulitz RC. Op. cit.

53. Brock TD. Op. cit:260.

54. Professor Robert Koch (obituary). Lancet 1910; 1:1583–8.

55. Daniel TM. Robert Koch, tuberculosis, and the subsequent history of medicine. Am Rev Resp Dis 1982; 125 (suppl):1–3.

Chapter 6: Pages 98-131

1. Daniel TM. Captain of death: The story of tuberculosis. Rochester, NY: University of Rochester Press, 1997.

2. Beagle FD. Health legislation. Thirty-sixth annual report of the State Health Department of New York for the year ending December 31, 1915. Volume 3. Albany, NY. 1916:139–48.

3. Winslow C-EA. The life of Hermann M. Biggs, M.D., D.Sc., LL.D. Physician and statesman of the public health. Philadelphia, PA: Lea & Febiger, 1929. This remarkable biography is notable because it was written by a colleague and close friend of Biggs and published only six years after Biggs's death. It a scholarly work written in an engaging style, and I have drawn upon it heavily for biographical material. A shorter biographical account is found in Walker MEM. Pioneers of public health. The story of some benefactors of the human race. New York: The Macmillan Company, 1930. Many obituaries were published in scientific journals at the time of Biggs death. Among them, biographical details are given in Hermann M. Biggs [obituary]. Science 1923; 58:413–5. A collection of tributes to Biggs following his death, which contain a number of insights into his life and personality, was published in Health News 1923; 18:160–84.

4. Winslow C-EA, 1929. Op. cit:22.

5. Ibid:24–29.

6. Bishop M. A history of Cornell. Ithaca, NY: Cornell University Press, 1962:41–2.

7. Ibid:61–2.

8. Heaton CE. A historical sketch of New York University College of Medicine 1841–1941. New York, NY: New York University, 1941.

9. Duffy J. The sanitarians. A history of American public health. Chicago, NY: University of Illinois Press, 1990. Chapter 12 of this scholarly and readable work deals with sanitary conditions in major American cities, including New York, at the time when Biggs enrolled in Medical School.

10. Winslow C-EA, 1929. Op. cit:39–43. Winslow quotes extensively from Biggs's thesis. The source is not cited, but Winslow had many Biggs family papers at his disposal.

11. Winslow C-EA, 1929. Op. cit:48–9.

12. At the time, sharp distinctions between clinical medicine and pathology did not exist, and, as in the days of Laennec, it was common for individuals interested in pathology to have clinical practices as well. Delafield was later to author with T. Mitchell Prudden, his friend and colleague, the first American text of pathology. Janeway was generally considered the finest diagnostician in New York, and he was the physi-

cian whom Edward Livingston Trudeau consulted when he developed symptoms of tuberculosis.

13. Winslow C-EA, 1929. Op. cit:65.

14. Biggs HM, Breneman AA. The epidemic of typhoid fever in Plymouth, Pa. NY Med J 1885; 41:576–9,637–9.

15. Both Bellevue Medical College and the College of Physicians and Surgeons were independent, proprietary medical schools at that time. Nonetheless, they were the preeminent medical schools of New York at that time. Bellevue Medical College merged with New York University Medical College in 1898 after a fire had destroyed its building. The College of Physicians and Surgeons became a part of Columbia University in 1891.

16. Anonymous. Biographical sketches and letters of T. Mitchell Prudden, M.D. New Haven, CT: Yale University Press, 1927. Although published anonymously, this book appears to have been chiefly assembled and edited by Prudden's sister, Lillian E. Prudden.

17. Biggs HM. The Koch comma-bacillus and its relation to Asiatic cholera. Medical News 1885; 47:226–33.

18. Winslow C-EA, 1929. Op. cit:79–81, 91–100; Anonymous. Op. cit:46, 82–3.

19. Biggs HM. History of the recent outbreak of epidemic cholera in New York. Am J Med Sc 1893; 105:63–72.

20. Garrison FH. An introduction to the history of medicine. Fourth edition. Philadelphia: W.B. Saunders Company, 1913:584.

21. Duffy J. Op. cit:195.

22. Anonymous. Op. cit:45.

23. Winslow C–EA, 1929. Op. cit:115.

24. Winslow C–EA, 1929. Op. cit:91. Duffy J. A history of public health in New York City 1886–1966. New York, NY: Russell Sage Foundation, 1974:645.

25. Biggs HM, Prudden TM, Loomis HP. Report on the prevention of pulmonary tuberculosis to the Board of Health of New York City, 1889. Reprinted in Winslow C–EA, 1929. Op. cit: Appendix II, 393–6.

26. Koch R. The Nobel lecture on how the fight against tuberculosis now stands. Lancet 1906; 1:1449–51. Riley RL, O'Grady F. Airborne

infection. Transmission and control. New York, NY: The Macmillan Company, 1961:9–10.

27. Riley RL, O'Grady F. Op. cit.

28. Daniel TM. Op. cit:121–4.

29. Daniel TM. Op. cit:87–96.

30. Bichloride of mercury.

31. Circular distributed by the New York City Department of Health, 1889. Reprinted in Winslow C-EA, 1929. Op. cit:87–8.

32. Chapman JS, Dyerly MD. Intrafamilial transmission of tuberculosis. Am Rev Respir Dis 1964; 90:48–60.

33. Teller ME. The tuberculosis movement. A public health campaign in the progressive era. New York, NY: Greenwood Press, 1988:70.

34. Biggs HM, Huddleston JH. The sanitary supervision of tuberculosis as practised by the New York City Board of Health. Am J Med Sc 1895; 109:17–27.

35. The health board and compulsory reports (editorial). Medical Record 1897; 51:126–7.

36. Winslow C-EA, 1929. Op. cit:139.

37. Winslow C-EA, 1929. Op. cit:135.

38. Biggs HM. Sanitary measures for the prevention of tuberculosis in New York City and their results. JAMA 1902; 39:1635–40.

39. Caldwell M. The last crusade. The war on consumption. 1862–1954. New York, NY: Atheneum, 1988:179.

40. Biggs HM, Bolduan CF. The tuberculosis campaign. Its influence on the methods of public health work generally. Department of Health of the City of New York Reprint Series No. 8, August 1913.

41. Winslow C-EA, 1929. Op. cit:178.

42. Winslow C-EA, 1929. Op. cit:179.

43. Daniel TM. Op. cit:178–94.

44. Daniel TM. Captain of death: The story of tuberculosis. Rochester, NY: University of Rochester Press, 1997:178–84.

45. Rothman SM. Living in the shadow of death. Tuberculosis and the social experience of illness in American history. New York, NY: BasicBooks, 1994:191–3. Lerner BH. Contagion and confinement. Controlling tuberculosis along the Skid Road. Baltimore, MD: The Johns Hopkins University Press, 1998:116–8.

46. Winslow C-EA, 1929. Op. cit:251–65. Winslow, who was one

of the colleagues whom Biggs recruited, recounts these events in a delightful fashion, drawing upon his personal memories and correspondence and clippings saved by Biggs's wife.

47. Thirty-fifth annual report of the State Health Department of New York for the year ending December 31, 1914. Volume 1. Albany, NY. 1916:15–7, 88–106. See also Winslow C-EA, 1929. Op. cit:264–6, which provides an anecdotal account of these events by one of Biggs's associates.

48. Thirty-fifth annual report of the State Health Department of New York for the year ending December 31, 1914. Volume 1. Op. cit:1.

49. Nicoll M Jr. Foreword. Health News 1923; 38:159–61.

50. Winslow C-EA. Health News 1923; 18:172–3.

51. Thirty-sixth annual report of the State Health Department of New York for the year ending December 31, 1915. Volume 1. Albany, NY. 1917:48–55.

52. Thirty-eighth annual report of the State Health Department of New York for the year ending December 31, 1917. Volume 1. Albany, NY. 1918:1–4.

53. Fortieth annual report of the State Health Department of New York for the year ending December 31, 1919. Volume 1. Albany, NY. 1920:279–93.

54. Forty-first annual report of the State Health Department of New York for the year ending December 31, 1920. Volume 1. Albany, NY. 1922:1–2.

55. Winslow C-EA, 1929. Op. cit:347.

56. Forty-third annual report of the State Health Department of New York for the year ending December 31, 1922. Volume 1. Albany, NY. 1923:1.

57. Ibid.

58. Biggs HM. Practical objectives in health work during the next twenty years. Health News 1923; 18:214–21.

59. Flexner S. Health News 1923; 18:166–7.

Chapter 7: Pages 132-155

1. For biographical information, I have relied principally on Wagner R. Clemens von Pirquet. His life and work. Baltimore, MD: The Johns

Hopkins Press, 1968. (Material from Wagner used with permission.) Wagner was von Pirquet's associate for more than a decade and his close friend. Additional biographical information (much of it obviously derived from Wagner) is available in: Rappaport HG. Clemens von Pirquet and allergy. Ann Allergy 1973; 31:467–75. Bendiner E. Baron von Pirquet: The aristocrat who discovered and defined allergy. Hosp Pract 1981; 16:137–58. Turk JL. Von Pirquet, allergy and infectious diseases: a review. J Royal Soc Med 1987; 80:31–3. Chick H. Clemens Pirquet and his work as director of the Vienna University Kinderklinik, 1911–1929. Lancet 1929; 1:624–6. Clemens Pirquet, M.D. [obituary]. Brit Med J 1929; 1:526. Clemens von Pirquet, M.D. 1874–1929 [obituary]. Am J Dis Child 1929; 37, 838–9. This final obituary was signed "B.S.," and one must suppose that it was written by Béla Schick.

2. Wagner R. Op. cit:23–4.

3. Rowntree LG. Amid masters of twentieth century medicine. Springfield, IL: Charles C. Thomas Publisher, 1958:166.

4. Kallós P. Introduction. Progress in Allergy 1:v–xiii, 1939. This volume of Progress in Allergy was reprinted in 1967, and the English language introduction quoted here was added in that republished edition. Used with permission.

5. The first anaphylactic fatality due to diphtheria antiserum occurred in 1896 in the daughter of Paul Langerhans, the noted pathologist. See Wagner R. Op. cit:57.

6. Wagner R. Op. cit:31.

7. Major RH. Classic descriptions of disease with biographical sketches of the authors. Springfield, IL: Charles C. Thomas, 1932:618–25.

8. Von Pirquet C. Allergie. Muenchener Med Wochenschrift 1906; 53:1457–8. This paper has been translated by a number of authors. I have used the translation of Wagner R. Op. cit:64–5.

9. Von Pirquet C. Allergy. Archives Internal Med 1911; 7:257–88, 383–436.

10. The use of tuberculin as a test for tuberculosis in children. Lancet 1909; 1:1612.

11. Von Pirquet C. Frequency of tuberculosis in childhood. JAMA 1909; 52:675–8. Copyright © 1909, American Medical Association. Used with permission.

12. Von Pirquet C. The relation of tuberculosis to infant mortality. New York Med J 1909; 40:1045–6. This paper was read two weeks before its publication at a Conference on the Prevention of Infant Mortality, New Haven, CT, November 17, 1909.

13. Von Pirquet C, 1909a. Op. cit.

14. Bett WR. Brit J Children's Dis 1929; 26:276–82.

15. Von Pirquet C, 1909b. Op. cit.

16. Von Pirquet C, 1909a. Op. cit.

17. Wagner R. Op. cit:77.

18. Bendiner E. Op. cit.

19. Von Pirquet CF. The importance of a thorough teaching of infectious diseases of childhood in the medical curriculum. Bull Med Chirug Faculty of Maryland 1910; 2:211–8.

20. Chesney AM. The Johns Hopkins Hospital and the Johns Hopkins University School of Medicine. A chronicle. Volume III. Baltimore, MD: The Johns Hopkins Press, 1963:106. The translation is used with permission.

21. Ibid:124.

22. Wagner R. Op. cit:87.

23. Chick H. Op. cit.

24. Wagner R. Op. cit:127.

25. Ibid:163.

26. Ibid:171.

Chapter 8: Pages 156-177

1. For biographic information about Frost I have relied chiefly on Maxcy KF. Papers of Wade Hampton Frost, M.D. A contribution to epidemiologic method. New York, NY: The Commonwealth Fund, 1941 and Gwaltney JM. Wade Hampton Frost, MD. A wider view of the world. Virginia Medical Quarterly 1995; 122:261–4. Other less comprehensive sources that I have consulted include: Dr. Wade Frost [obituary]. Lancet 1938; 1:1252; Merrell M. The Reed-Frost collaboration. Am J Epidemiol 1976; 104:364–9; Sartwell PE. The contributions of Wade Hampton Frost. Am J Epidemiol 1976; 104:386–91; Stebbins EL. Wade Hampton Frost: An appreciation. Am J Epidemiol 1976;

104:392–5; Terris M. The epidemiologic tradition. The Wade Hampton Frost lecture. Public Health Reports 1979; 94:203–9; Lilienfeld AM. Wade Hampton Frost: Contributions to epidemiology and public health. Am J Epidemiol 1983; 117:379–83; and Comstock GW. Invited commentary on "the age selection mortality from tuberculosis in successive decades." Am J Epidemiol 1995; 141:3. Further information, including a number of personal details not available in published sources, were provided to me by Jack M. Gwaltney, M.D., Wade Hampton Frost Professor of Medicine, University of Virginia.

2. Schweiger BB. Putting politics aside: Virginia Democrats and voter apathy in the era of disfranchisement. In Ayers EL, Willis JC. The edge of the South. Life in nineteenth-century Virginia. Charlottesville, VA: University Press of Virginia, 1991:194–218.

3. Blanton WB. Medicine in Virginia in the nineteenth century. Richmond, VA: Garrett and Massie, Inc, 1933:98.

4. Mullan F. Plagues and politics: The story of the United States Public Health Service. New York: Basic Books, 1989:14.

5. Frost WH. An organism (*Pseudomonas protea*) isolated from water, agglutinated by the serum of typhoid fever patients. Hygienic Laboratory Bulletin 1910; 66:29–75; Frost WH. Note on an organism isolated from Washington tap water, agglutinated readily by the serum of typhoid fever patients. Am J Public Hygiene 1910; 6:670–1. Both of these reports are cited in the bibliography published by Maxcy KF. Op. cit:613.

6. Frost WH. The water supply of Williamson, West Virginia, and its relation to an epidemic of typhoid fever. Hygienic Laboratory Bulletin. 1910: 72:55–90. Reprinted in Maxcy KF. Op. cit:26–69.

7. Ibid:34–5. It should be noted that at that time most Americans did not expect municipal water systems to provide potable water.

8. Frost WH. The sewage pollution of streams; its relation to public health. Public Health Reports 1916; 31:2486–97. Reprinted in Maxcy KF. Op. cit:287–301.

9. Frost WH. A review of the work of the United States Public Health Service in investigations of stream pollution. Public Health Reports 1926; 41:75–85. Reprinted in Maxcy KF. Op. cit:302–15.

10. Daniel TM, Robbins FC. Polio. Rochester, NY: University of Rochester Press, 1997.

11. Frost WH. Epidemiologic studies of acute anterior poliomyelitis. Hygienic Laboratory Bulletin 1913; 90:9–105,234–52. Reprinted in Maxcy KF. Op. cit:120–269.

12. Frost WH. Statistics of influenza morbidity, with special reference to certain factors in case incidence and case fatality. Public Health Reports 1920; 35:584–97. Reprinted in Maxcy KF. Op. cit:340–58.

13. Frost WH. The epidemiology of influenza. JAMA 1919; 73:313–8. Reprinted in Maxcy KF. Op. cit:321–39.

14. Frost WH, 1920. Op. cit.

15. A delightful and informative account of the collaboration of Frost and Reed is provided by Merrell M. Op. cit.

16. Maxcy KF. Op. cit:617–8.

17. Brailey ME. Tuberculosis in white and negro children. Volume II. The epidemiologic aspects of the Harriet Lane study. Cambridge, MA: Harvard University Press, 1958.

18. Maxcy KF. Op. cit:617.

19. Frost WH. Risk of persons in familial contact with pulmonary tuberculosis. Amer J Public Health and the Nation's Health 1933; 23:426–32. Reprinted in Maxcy KF. Op. cit:582–92. Used with permission.

20. Ibid.

21. Zeidberg LD, Gass RS, Dillon A, Hutcheson RH. The Williamson County tuberculosis study. A twenty-four-year epidemiologic study. Am Rev Respir Dis 1963; 87(suppl):1–88. Official Journal of the American Thoracic Society. Copyright © American Lung Association. Used with permission.

22. Ibid:6.

23. Ibid:8–9.

24. Frost WH. How much control of tuberculosis? Amer J Public Health and the Nation's Health 1937; 27:759–66. Reprinted in Maxcy KF. Op. cit:601–12.

25. May RM. Ecology and population biology. In Warren KS, Mahmoud AAF, editors. Tropical and geographical medicine. Second edition. New York, NY: McGraw-Hill Information Services Company, 1990:130–45.

26. Frost WH. The age selection of mortality from tuberculosis in successive decades. Amer J Hygiene 1939; 30:91–6. Reprinted in Maxcy

KF. Op. cit:593–600. Reprinted in Amer J Epid 1995; 141:4–9. Material used with permission of APHA.

27. Ibid.

28. Ibid.

29. Frost WH, 1939. Op. cit.

30. King Henry the Fourth—Part One: act 2, scene 3, line 108. William Shakespeare. The Complete Works. London: Collins, 1951.

Chapter 9: Pages 178-201

1. Waksman SA. My life with the microbes. New York, NY: Simon and Schuster, 1954. Used with permission.

2. Ibid. This autobiography has been my chief source for information about the life of Waksman, especially during his early years. Similarly, all biographers of Waksman have used this book as their principal source. It was written when he was in his mid sixties. Later chapters recounting his travels were obviously taken from journals kept during these trips, but the accounts of his early life must certainly reflect the personal biases that creep into the distant recollections of every person. Much autobiographical material is also contained in Waksman SA. The conquest of tuberculosis. Berkeley, CA: University of California Press, 1964. Additional details of Waksman's life are provided by Sakula A. Selman Waksman (1888–1973), discoverer of streptomycin: A centenary review. Brit J Dis Chest 1988; 82:23–31, 137.

3. Waksman SA, 1954. Op. cit:17–8.

4. Ibid:39–40.

5. Waksman SA, Curtis RE. The actinomyces of the soil. Soil Science 1916; 1:99–134. This paper is reproduced in Woodruff HB (editor). Scientific contributions of Selman A. Waksman. Selected articles published in honor of his 80th birthday July 22, 1968. New Brunswick, NJ: Rutgers University Press:11–53.

6. Warren JV. Jokichi Takamine (1854–1922). J Lab Clin Med 1988; 112:793–4.

7. Waksman SA. Principles of soil microbiology. Baltimore, MD: Williams & Wilkins Co, 1927.

8. Woodruff HB (editor), 1968. Op. cit:xx.

9. Waksman SA, Curtis RE. Op. cit.

10. Ibid:119.

11. Waksman SA, Henrici, AT. The nomenclature and classification of the actinomycetes. J Bacteriol 1943; 46:337–41. This paper is reproduced in Woodruff HB (editor), 1968:225–30.

12. Waksman SA, 1954. Op. cit:129.

13. Ibid:145.

14. Ibid. Chapter 13.

15. Ackernecht EH. A short history of medicine. Revised edition. Baltimore, MD: The Johns Hopkins University Press, 1982:232–3. Waksman SA, Woodruff HB. The soil as a source of microorganisms antagonistic to disease-producing bacteria. J Bacteriol 1940; 40:581–600. This paper (pages 137–56) is reproduced in Woodruff HB (editor), 1968. Op. cit:257–76.

16. Waksman SA, Starkey RL. Partial sterilization of soil, microbiological activities and soil fertility. Soil Sc 1923; 16:137–56, 247–68, 343–57. The first section of this paper (pages 137–56) is reproduced in Woodruff HB (editor), 1968. Op. cit:77–97.

17. Waksman SA, Foster JW. Associative and antagonistic effects of microorganisms: II. Antagonistic effects of microorganisms grown on artificial substrates. Soil Science 1937; 43:69–76. Reproduced in Woodruff HB (editor), 1968. Op. cit:249–56.

18. Waksman SA, 1954. Op. cit:211–3.

19. Ibid:261.

20. Dubos R, Dubos J. The white plague. Tuberculosis, man, and society. Boston, MA: Little, Brown, and Company, 1952.

21. Farber S. Opening remarks. Cancer Chemotherapy Reports 1974; 58:5–7.

22. Waksman SA, 1954. Op. cit:231.

23. Waksman SA, Woodruff HB. Selective antibiotic action of various substances of microbial origin. J Bacteriol 1942; 44:373–84.

24. Waksman SA. Antagonistic relations of microorganisms. Bacteriol Rev 1941; 5:231–91. Waksman SA. What is an antibiotic or an antibiotic substance? Mycologia 1947; 39:565–9.

25. Waksman SA. Letter to the editor. Amer Scientist 1953; 41:8,10,12. Burkholder PR. Comments by Dr. Burkholder. Amer Scientist 1953; 41:12,14.

26. Waksman SA, 1953. Op. cit.

27. Waksman SA. Quoted by Comroe JH Jr. Pay dirt: the story of streptomycin. Part I. From Waksman to Waksman. Am Rev Respir Dis 1978; 117:773–81. Comroe's article, including the companion paper (Pay dirt: the story of streptomycin. Part II. Feldman and Hinshaw; Lehman. Am Rev Respir Dis 1978; 117:957–968), provides an excellent account of the history of the discovery of streptomycin.

28. Waksman SA, 1954. Op. cit:232–3.

29. Waksman SA, 1964. Op. cit:103–4. Comroe JH Jr. Retrospectroscope. Menlo Park, CA: Von Gehr Press, 1977:71.

30. Ryan F. The forgotten plague. How the battle against tuberculosis was won—and lost. Boston, MA: Little, Brown and Company, 1992.

31. Two years later, the Nobel Prize in Medicine or Physiology was awarded to John Enders, Thomas Weller, and Frederick Robbins for the cultivation of the poliovirus. Weller and Robbins were postdoctoral fellows in Enders's laboratory, and this appears to have been the first time that junior laboratory workers were included in the award. In this case, Enders had repeatedly described the work as a team effort, specifically noting the contributions of Weller and Robbins, and the Noble committee made intensive, although covert, investigations to document the contributions of Robbins and Weller (personal conversations with Frederick C. Robbins).

32. Daniel TM. Captain of death: The story of tuberculosis. Rochester, NY: University of Rochester Press, 1997:201–14. Ryan F. Op. cit. Waksman SA, 1964. Op. cit:103–18. Comroe JH Jr, 1978. Op. cit.

33. Schatz A, Bugie E, Waksman SA. Streptomycin, a substance exhibiting antibiotic activity against Gram-positive and Gram-negative bacteria. Proc Soc Exptl Biol Med 1944; 55:66–9.

34. Schatz A, Waksman SA. Effect of streptomycin and other antibiotic substances upon *Mycobacterium tuberculosis* and related organisms. Proc Soc Exptl Biol Med 1944; 57:244–8.

35. Waksman SA, Bugie E, Schatz A. Isolation of antibiotic substances from soil micro-organisms, with special reference to streptothricin and streptomycin. Proc Staff Meetings of the Mayo Clinic 1944; 19:537–48. Waksman SA, Schatz A. Streptomycin—origin, nature, and properties. J Amer Pharmaceut Assoc 1945; 34:273–91.

36. Ryan F. Op. cit:235.

37. Feldman WH. Streptomycin: Some historical aspects of its development as a chemotherapeutic agent in tuberculosis. Amer Rev Tuberc 1954; 69:859–68.

38. Daniel TM. Op. cit:210–12. Ryan F. Op. cit:237–9.

39. Ryan F. Op. cit:332–9. This well researched account contrasts with that of Waksman SA, 1954. Op. cit:279–85. Ryan's account is based on interviews with Schatz and documents preserved by Schatz. They may have been biased. Waksman's account was based on his recollections and documents, also perhaps biased.

40. Woodruff HB (editor). Op. cit:365–9.

41. Ibid:287–305.

42. Waksman SA, 1954. Op. cit:358–9.

Chapter 10: Pages 205-209

v1. Banting FG, Best CH. The internal secretion of the pancreas. J Lab Clin Med 1922; 7:465–80.

v2. Ten great public health achievements—United States, 1900–1999. MMWR 1999; 48:241–3.

3. Fudenberg HH. The dollar benefits of biomedical research: A cost analysis. J Lab Clin Med 1988; 111:6–12.

4. Murray CJL, Dejonghe E, Chum HJ, Nyangulu DS, Salomao A, Styblo K. Cost effectiveness of chemotherapy for pulmonary tuberculosis in three sub-Saharan African countries. Lancet 1991; 338:1305–8.

Glossary

Medical and Technical Terms
Used in This Books

Acquired immunodeficiency syndrome. A disease of the human immune system caused by a virus and commonly known by its acronym, AIDS.

Actinomyces. A genus of microorganisms native to the soil that yielded many early antibiotics.

Actinomyces griseus. Original name for Streptomyces griseus, the organism from which streptomycin was isolated.

Actinomycete. A general term for any one of the members of the genus Actinomyces and closely related organisms.

Actinomycin. An antibiotic derived from actinomycetes. The first such antibiotic found by Waksman. Too toxic for use in treating infections, it has seen some use as a chemotherapeutic agent for treating cancer.

Active tuberculosis. Tuberculosis in its active state as defined by the presence of living tubercle bacilli or changing diseases process within the preceding six months.

Adrenocortical steroids. Hormones secreted by the adrenal glands, including cortisone, which are capable of immunosuppression. Often used in the treatment of allergic or rheumatic diseases.

Aesclepiads. Early society of Greek physicians on the Island of Kos.

AIDS. Acronym and common name for the acquired immunodeficiency syndrome.

Allergen. An antigen inducing an allergic response, especially common nasal allergies.

Allergy. A state of altered reactivity to a precipitating agent, which is known as an antigen or allergen.

American Lung Association. Originally the National Association for the Study and Prevention of Tuberculosis, the oldest voluntary health agency, widely known for its Christmas seals.

American Society for Microbiology. The largest American professional society of microbiologists. Originally the Society of American Bacteriologists.

American Thoracic Society. The largest American professional society of medical doctors specializing in pulmonary diseases. Originally the American Sanatorium Association and later the American Trudeau Society.

Aminoglycoside. The chemical class of antibiotics that includes streptomycin, neomycin, and others.

Anamnestic response. An accelerated and augmented response to an antigen upon second or reexposure to the antigen.

Anergy. Paradoxical absence of an immune response.

Angioneurotic edema. A potentially severe allergic reaction characterized by swelling of the face, tongue, and vocal cords.

Anthrax. A disease of grazing animals and occasionally humans caused by *Bacillus anthracis.*

Antibiotic. A substance produced by a microorganism that is capable of arresting the growth of or killing other microorganisms.

Antibody. A protein in the blood serum that is induced by contact with and subsequently capable of reacting specifically with foreign substances, which are termed antigens.

Antigen. A foreign substance capable of inducing the formation of and reacting specifically with antibodies or sensitized lymphocytes.

Antiserum. Serum containing antibodies from the blood of a person or animal containing antibodies.

Arrested tuberculosis. Tuberculosis that no longer shows signs of activity—that is, is unchanging and no longer a source of living tubercle bacilli. Prior to the introduction of antibiotic therapy, tuberculosis was thought never to be cured, and the term arrested designated a currently healed state of disease that nevertheless was still thought to be capable of reactivating.

Asepsis. Literally, without infection. This term is used to designate the exclusion of microorganisms.

Attenuated. Literally, drawn out. This term is used to describe microorganisms that have become altered to be less virulent or nonvirulent for humans.

Auscultation. Literally, the act of listening. In medicine, the act of examination by listening to a body organ or system.

Bacille Calmette-Guérin. An attenuated strain of *Mycobacterium bovis* developed by Calmette and Guérin as a vaccine against tuberculosis.

Bacillus. This term is commonly used generically to describe microorganisms and as a synonym for bacterium. More narrowly defined, it refers specifically to members of the genus Bacillus, long, thin bacteria with specific growth, reproductive, and staining characteristics.

Bactericidal. An adjective used to describe drugs capable of killing bacteria.

Bacteriological. Of or pertaining to bacteriology.

Bacteriology. The science or study of bacteria.

Bacteriostatic. An adjective used to describe drugs capable of halting the growth of but not killing bacteria.

Bacterium. A term commonly used to designated a type of single-celled microorganism, including many that produce disease.

B-cell. A colloquial designation for B-lymphocyte.

BCG. The acronym and colloquial term for Bacille Calmette-Guérin, a vaccine against tuberculosis.

B-lymphocyte. A class of lymphocyte specialized for the production of antibody.

Booster response. Anamnestic response.

Bronchiectasis. A destructive disease of the lungs in which small respiratory bronchioles end in saccules. Usually associated with repeated infection and hemoptysis.

Bronchitis. Irritation or infection of a bronchus or of bronchi.

Bronchus. A tubular airway, a series of which connect the trachea (wind pipe) with the lungs.

Captain of Death. Sobriquet for tuberculosis from John Bunyan's *The Life and Death of Mr. Badman.*

Cavity. A hole or vacant space within an area of diseased tissue and a result of the disease process. Similar to an abscess, but usually used in conjunction with processes such as tuberculosis that are more chronic in nature than diseases associated with abscesses.

CD4+ T-lymphocyte. A subclass of T-lymphocytes responsible for immunologic memory and promoting cellular immune responses. These cells are recognizable by surface antigens that can be identified with appropriate antisera.

Cellular Immunity. Immunity mediated by cells, specifically by T-lymphocytes.

Centers for Disease Control and Prevention. An agency of the United States Public Health Service responsible for both control programs and research on diseases of public health concern in the United States. Frequently referred to by the acronym "CDC."

Chemotherapy. The treatment of disease with chemical agents. While this term is most commonly known today as a form of cancer treatment, the term is also applied to the treatment of tuberculosis with drugs.

Cholera. A fulminant, often fatal diarrheal disease caused by *Vibrio cholera.*

Cirrhosis of the liver, Laennec's. A scarring of the liver associated with excessive alcohol consumption. Although not originally described by him, Laennec's name is associated with this condition because of his elegant description of it.

Cohort. An epidemiological term used to designate a group of individuals sharing one or more defining common characteristics.

Conidia. A fungal spore.

Consumption. An older term for tuberculosis.

Cytokine. A substance produced by one cell and capable of reacting with and inducing responses in other cells of the same or different types. This term is usually reserved for substances and cells of the immune system.

Delayed hypersensitivity. A type of immune response mediated by specific lymphocytes and characterized by an onset delayed by one or two days after reexposure to the inciting antigen. This type of hypersensitivity is characteristic of tuberculosis.

Diphtheria. A severe, often fatal type of pharyngitis.

DNA. The acronym and colloquial name for deoxyribose nucleic acid. Genes are composed of specific configurations of this complex molecule.

DNA Library. Multiple fragments of the genome of an organism placed into the genome of another convenient organism, usually *Escheri-*

chia coli, in such a fashion that the other organism will express the genes of the first and synthesize the products for which those genes code, thus facilitating their study.

Egophony. Also called haegophonism by Laennec. A change in the character of sound transmitted through the lungs and chest so that they take on a bleating sound, a long e typically sounding like a long a.

Emphysema. A condition of the lungs in which the air spaces become enlarged by destruction of the fine septae between them. Clinically it is manifested by severe shortness of breath.

Epidemic. Literally, upon a people. An outbreak of disease in a population.

Epidemiologist. A scientist trained to study epidemics.

Epidemiology. The science of the study of epidemics.

Escherichia coli. A bacterium widespread in nature, especially in the colon. Most strains are not pathogenic; some secrete toxins and cause diarrheal disease.

Etiology. The cause of a disease or pathological condition.

Extrapulmonary. Outside of the lungs. Used as extrapulmonary tuberculosis to describe tuberculosis occurring in other parts of the body.

Fomes, fomites (plural). Strictly defined, any inanimate object or particle capable of transmitting infection by absorbing germs onto and transmitting them from its surface. Generally used to refer to sedentary particles rather than airborne particles.

Gene. That portion of DNA encoding for a particular trait, often for a single protein.

Genome. The entire assembly of genetic material of an organism. Present as DNA within chromosomes.

Genus. A taxonomic term used to designate a group of related species of organisms. By convention, genus names are always written out when first used in a text and capitalized and italicized, but thereafter may be abbreviated with the first letter only followed by a period.

Ghon complex. A healed peripheral lung nodule and regional lymph node visible on a chest radiograph. This complex often represents the healed residuum of primary tuberculosis.

Gramicidin. An antibiotic isolated by René Dubos and used for topical treatment of wound infections.

Granuloma. An immunologically mediated tissue inflammatory response typical of delayed hypersensitivity reactions. The characteristic tissue response to tuberculosis.

Hemoptysis. The coughing of blood.

HIV. An acronym for human immunodeficiency virus.

Human immunodeficiency virus. The virus that causes the acquired immunodeficiency syndrome (AIDS).

Hygiene. The science of health maintenance and disease prevention.

Hypersensitivity. An altered state of reactivity with increased responses. This term is typically applied to allergic responses.

Hypochondrium. The area of the abdomen just below (hypo) the ribs (chondria).

Immune. Classically, this term means resistant to infection or disease. In modern usage, this term is often limited to the case where the resistance is acquired and is mediated by specific, antigen-induced, lymphocyte or antibody-mediated host responses.

Immunity. The state or condition of being immune. There are two types of immunity, that mediated by serum antibodies and that mediated by T lymphocytes.

Immunochemistry. The science of reactions involving immunoglobulins.

Immunodeficiency. A lack of immunity under circumstances where immunity would ordinarily exist.

Immunoglobulin. A member of the class of serum proteins that includes antibodies. Immunoglobulins are further classified as immunoglobulin-G, -M, -A, -E, and -D.

Immunologist. A scientist trained to study immunity.

Immunology. The science of the study of immunity.

Immunosuppression. The state of or act of suppression of immunity.

Inactive tuberculosis. Tuberculosis showing no current signs of activity.

Incidence. The rate of occurrence of a disease or a condition within a specified period of time. Often expressed for tuberculosis as the number of new cases per one hundred thousand population per year.

Index case. The first case of a disease or condition identified in investigating an epidemic or outbreak.

Influenza. A viral disease with prominent bronchitis that often occurs in epidemics.

Inoculate. To impart by injection, as to introduce a microorganism into culture medium, or as to inject a vaccine.

Isoniazid. Isonicotinic acid hydrazide. A bactericidal drug used for the treatment of tuberculosis.

Lupus vulgaris. Tuberculosis of the skin. An archaic dermatologic term not commonly used today.

Lymph. Fluid in lymphatic channels originating as extracellular fluid in tissues. This term was used by Koch to describe the fluid phase of his cultures of tubercle bacilli.

Lymphatic. Thin-walled vessel that drains lymph from the body, eventually returning it to the venous system.

Lymphocyte. The class of white blood cells that includes cells with immunologic functions, including immunologic memory.

Lymphokine. A cytokine produced by lymphocytes.

M. bovis. Shortened form of *Mycobacterium bovis.*

M. tuberculosis. Shortened form of *Mycobacterium tuberculosis.*

Macrophage. A large white blood cell and tissue cell capable of ingesting materials and particles foreign to the host. This cell participates in cellular (delayed) immune responses. It is the principal cell present in granulomas. When circulating in the blood, it is usually known as a monocyte.

Mediate auscultation. Auscultation performed with an instrument, such as a stethoscope, placed between the examiner's ear and the patient.

Microbe. A bacterium or germ. A microorganism.

Microbiologist. A scientist trained in the study of microorganisms.

Microbiology. The science of the study of microorganisms.

Microorganism. An organism or life form too small to be seen without the aid of a microscope, such as a microbe.

Miliary tubercles. Small, disseminated tubercles characteristic of miliary tuberculosis.

Miliary tuberculosis. Tuberculosis that has spread through the blood stream to seed all organs of the body. The term miliary originated with early pathologists performing autopsies on tuberculosis patients who noted that the small granulomas or tubercles in the lungs looked like millet seeds.

Molecular biology. The study of biological phenomena, especially the study of genetic events, at the molecular level.

Monocyte. A large white blood cell that enters tissues to participate in immune responses. In tissues it is known as a macrophage.

Mycelium. The filamentous part of a fungal colony.

Mycobacteriophage. A phage specific for mycobacteria.

Mycobacterium. The genus of bacteria that includes the tubercle bacillus and related species. By convention, genus names are always written out when first used in a text and capitalized but thereafter may be abbreviated with the first letter only followed by a period (*M.*).

Mycobacterium bovis. The bovine type of tubercle bacillus. It causes disease in cattle and also in many other mammals including humans.

Mycobacterium tuberculosis. The scientific name for the tubercle bacillus. The bacterium that causes tuberculosis.

Mycobacterium ulcerans. The member of the genus *Mycobacterium* that causes Buruli or Bairnsdale ulcer, a chronic skin disease seen in certain tropical areas.

Mycobacterium vaccae. A nonpathogenic mycobacterium proposed as a vaccine to enhance immunity for use as an adjuvant to chemotherapy for the treatment of tuberculosis.

National Association for the Study and Prevention of Tuberculosis. Original name for the National Tuberculosis Association, in turn later renamed the American Lung Association.

National Institutes of Health. An agency of the United States Public Health Service responsible for research on disease and disease processes. Often known by the acronym NIH.

National Tuberculosis Association. A voluntary health agency devoted to fighting tuberculosis. Name changed and later became the American Lung Association.

Neomycin. An antibiotic of the aminoglycoside category, which also includes streptomycin.

Nidation. Literally, nesting. The process of becoming established in the body by a microorganism.

Parenchyma. The tissue of an organ.

Pathogenic. Capable of causing disease.

Pathogenesis. The evolution of a disease process as related to its cause.

Pathology. An abnormality of an organ or tissue, often associated with disease in that organ or tissue. The science and study of such abnormalities and of pathogenesis.

PCR. Acronym for polymerase chain reaction.

Pebrine. An infectious disease of silk worms.

Pectoriloquy. Also called pectorlioquism by Laennec. A change in the character of sounds transmitted through the lungs and chest so that they appear to originate very close to the ear.

Penicillin. An antibiotic of the beta-lactam category.

Percussion. Literally, the act of hitting or striking. In medicine, examination by tapping an area or organ and perceiving the resonance generated from the impact.

Peritonitis. An infection of the lining of the abdominal cavity.

Phage. A virus capable of infecting bacteria.

Phagocyte. A cell capable of phagocytosis.

Phagocytosis. The act of ingestion by a cell.

Phlebotomy. Literally, the act of making a hole in a vein. The withdrawal of blood as a form of medical treatment or, in modern usage, to obtain blood samples for diagnostic testing.

Phthisis. The ancient Greek word for tuberculosis. It remained in use in medical terminology well through the nineteenth century. It was generally used to refer to pulmonary tuberculosis.

Plague. A disease of the lymph nodes and sometimes lungs that has caused major epidemics, including the Black Death, and for which fleas on rats act as a vector, transporting it from place to place.

Plasmid. Genetic material in bacteria located within the cytoplasm outside of the cell nucleus.

Pleura. The membrane lining the chest cavity and covering the surfaces of the lungs.

Pleurisy. Inflammation of the pleura.

Pleurisy with effusion. Pleurisy accompanied by the accumulation of fluid in the pleural space. A common manifestation of tuberculosis, especially primary tuberculosis.

Polymerase chain reaction. A chemical reaction conveniently carried out under laboratory conditions by which DNA reproduces itself in large numbers. This reaction facilitates the study of DNA and genes.

Postprimary tuberculosis. Tuberculosis developing directly after the primary infection without an initial healing. Also called progressive postprimary tuberculosis.

Pott's disease. Tuberculous spondylitis. This disease was first described by Percival Pott.

PPD. Purified protein derivative of tuberculin.

Precipitin reaction. The reaction of antibody with antigen in a test tube to produce a visible precipitate.

Prevalence. The amount of disease present in a population at any given time usually expressed as a ratio, fraction, or percent, often for tuberculosis as number of cases per one hundred thousand.

Primary tuberculosis. Tuberculosis occurring directly following initial infection with tubercle bacilli. The first tuberculosis disease episode. Often a mild and unnoticed illness with spontaneous remission.

Prontosil. A red dye found to be bacteriostatic for many bacteria. Its active moiety was sulfanilamide, the first sulfonamide drug.

Public health. The discipline of health maintenance and disease prevention applied using measures applicable to communities or populations.

Public Health Service, United States. A uniformed service of the United States responsible for the health of the nation.

Puerperal sepsis. Infection of the female genital tract associated with obstetrical delivery.

Pulmonary. Of or relating to the lungs.

Purified protein derivative. A material prepared from tuberculin that is semipurified and more readily standardized than crude tuberculin. The material commonly used for tuberculin testing today.

Quarantine. Isolation or exclusion by law of infected individuals in order to prevent disease transmission.

Reactivation tuberculosis. Tuberculosis that has become inactive and again become active.

Rinderpest. A viral disease of cattle enzootic in southern Africa.

Salvarsan. An arsenical chemotherapeutic agent discovered by Ehrlich. Effective for the treatment of trypanosomiasis and syphilis. The first specific chemotherapeutic agent.

Sanatorium. A hospital or health facility providing treatment for chronic disease, especially tuberculosis. Sometimes, used synonymously with sanitarium. Sanitorium is used throughout this book, except in referring to the Adirondack Cottage Sanitarium, founded by Trudeau and named thus by him.

Sanitarium. A term often used synonymously with sanatorium. Originally, sanitarium meant a spa or facility for general health promotion, but not an institution for specific treatment of diseases.

Scarlatina. Scarlet fever.

Scarlet fever. A disease with a skin rash that follows streptococcal pharyngitis.

Scrofula. Tuberculosis of the lymph nodes in the neck. The term derives from a Latin word meaning little pig or suckling sow. The swelling produced in the neck was said to cause children with scrofula to have a neck like that of a pig.

Sepsis. Infection, often used to connote generalized infection with pathogenic microorganisms in the blood stream.

Serum. The liquid phase of clotted blood. Sometimes used synonymously with antiserum.

Serum sickness. An allergic disease caused by reaction to a foreign protein, especially horse serum used for treating certain diseases such as diphtheria and tetanus.

Simon foci. Silent, quiescent, microscopic foci in the apical portions of the lung that are thought to be the progenitors of active tuberculosis at those sites.

Society of American Bacteriologists. Original name for the American Society for Microbiology.

Species. A taxonomic group of organisms sufficiently closely related so as to be considered of a single type. By convention, species names are not abbreviated and are not capitalized.

Spore. The reproductive unit of some microbes, analogous to seeds of plants. Spores are usually hardy and resist most extremes of environmental conditions.

Sputum. Respiratory secretions.

Staphylococcus. A genus of bacteria, many species of which are pathogenic and commonly associated with sound and skin infections.

Stethoscope. A medical instrument used for auscultation.

Streptococcus. A genus of bacteria, may species of which are pathogenic and commonly associated with pharyngeal or respiratory infections, including pneumonia.

Streptomyces. A genus of microorganisms, most of which are soil organisms.

Streptomyces griseus. The soil microbe from which streptomycin was isolated.

Streptomycin. An antibiotic isolated from *Streptomyces griseus* by Selman Waksman and Albert Schatz. It is bactericidal for tubercle bacilli.

TB. Colloquial term for tuberculosis.

T-cell. A colloquial designation for T-lymphocyte.

Thiacetazone. Thioacetazone.

Thioacetazone. A semithiocarbazone drug that is bacteriostatic against tubercle bacilli. Not used in the United States. Widely used in developing countries because of its low cost.

Tibione. Trade name for thioacetazone.

T-lymphocyte. A lymphocyte named for its relation to the thymus gland and responsible for immunologic memory and mediation of delayed hypersensitivity reactions.

Trachea. The central windpipe. The airway beginning at the larynx and connecting the mouth and nose with bronchi leading to the lungs.

Transposon. A fragment of DNA capable of moving to other locations in the genome and replicating into multiple copies. Also termed an insertion sequence. Sometimes called a "jumping gene."

Trypanosomiasis. An encephalitis of cattle and occasionally humans commonly known as "African Sleeping Sickness."

Tubercle. A granuloma due to tuberculosis.

Tubercle bacillus. A colloquial term for *Mycobacterium tuberculosis*, the microbe that causes tuberculosis.

Tubercular. Strictly defined, an adjective meaning having tubercles. Commonly, and in a strict sense incorrectly, used as a synonym for tuberculous.

Tuberculin. The sterile filtrate of liquid cultures of tubercle bacilli. It contains many antigens of tubercle bacilli and is injected in small quantities as a diagnostic aid for identifying individuals infected with tubercle bacilli.

Tuberculin purified protein derivative. Purified protein derivative, PPD.

Tuberculin skin test. Tuberculin test.

Tuberculin test. A test in which a small amount of dilute tuberculin or PPD is introduced into the skin. A reaction to the introduced antigen is termed a positive tuberculin test and indicates prior infection with the tubercle bacillus.

Tuberculosis. The chronic, wasting disease caused by *Mycobacterium tuberculosis* or *M. bovis.*

Tuberculous. An adjective meaning having tuberculosis or related to tuberculosis.

Tuberculous meningitis. Tuberculosis of the meninges, the membranes covering the brain.

Tuberculous spondylitis. Tuberculosis of the spine.

Typhoid fever. An infectious disease of the intestinal tract caused by *Salmonella typhi.*

Variolation. The practice of cutaneous inoculation of infective smallpox (variola) material with the intent of producing a local skin lesion that would confer immunity against smallpox.

Vector. An agent responsible for transmitting an infection but not itself pathogenic.

Vibrio cholera. The bacterium that causes cholera.

Virulence. The capacity of a microorganism to produce disease.

Virulent. Possessing virulence.

Vitreous humor. The transparent liquid within the eye.

White Plague. A descriptive term for tuberculosis. while the term had prior usage, it was popularized by René and Jean Dubos with its inclusion in the title of their book, The White Plague—Tuberculosis, Man, and Society.

Woods Hole Oceanographic Institute. A research institute in Wood Hole, Massachusetts with major laboratories for the study of marine biology.

Yellow fever. A viral disease transmitted by mosquitos, named because jaundice is a usual feature.

Yersinia pestis. The bacterium that causes plague.

Index

Throughout history, tuberculosis has been at or near the top of the list of infectious diseases that have plagued humankind. This pervasive disease has had a central position not only in causing illness but also in challenging medical scientists to understand it—and, in so doing, to further understand all of human health and illness. *Pioneers in Medicine and Their Impact on Tuberculosis* tells the stories of six of these individuals: Rene Theophile Hyacinthe Laennec (pathology), Heinrich Hermann Robert Koch (bacteriology), Hermann Michael Biggs (public health), Clemens von Pirquet (immunology), Wade Hampton Frost (epidemiology), and Selman Abraham Waksman (antiobiotics). It examines not only their contributions in their own fields but their special work in conquering tuberculosis. Presenting their fascinating lives and the seminal work they did in their disciplines, the author examines the importance of their discoveries and relates them to the dramatic expansion of medical science during the era in which they lived.

THOMAS M. DANIEL is Professor Emeritus of Medicine and International Health; he is Emeritus Director of the Center for International Health at Case Western Reserve University. His previous book, *Captain of Death: The Story of Tuberculosis* (University of Rochester Press, 1997) was "strongly recommended" by the *New England Journal of Medicine*, and was selected by *Choice* for its Outstanding Academic Book List for 1998.